THE **Healthy Smoothie** Bible

THE **Healthy Smoothie** Bible

Lose Weight, Detoxify, Fight Disease, and Live Long

Farnoosh Brock

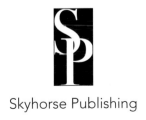

Skyhorse Publishing

Skyhorse Publishing books may be purchased in bulk at special discounts for sales promotion, corporate gifts, fund-raising, or educational purposes. Special editions can also be created to specifications. For details, contact the Special Sales Department, Skyhorse Publishing, 307 West 36th Street, 11th Floor, New York, NY 10018 or info@skyhorsepublishing.com.

Skyhorse® and Skyhorse Publishing® are registered trademarks of Skyhorse Publishing, Inc.®, a Delaware corporation.

Visit our website at www.skyhorsepublishing.com.

10 9 8 7 6 5

Library of Congress Cataloging-in-Publication Data is available on file.

ISBN: 978–1-62873-712-7

Printed in China

Disclaimer

This book is not meant to be used to diagnose or treat any medical condition. For diagnosis or treatment of any medical problem, consult your own physician. Consult with your doctor before beginning any new diet or exercise regimen.

For more information about smoothies, please visit:
http://www.prolificjuicing.com/healthysmoothies

To all who seek health and healing from Mother Nature

Table of Contents

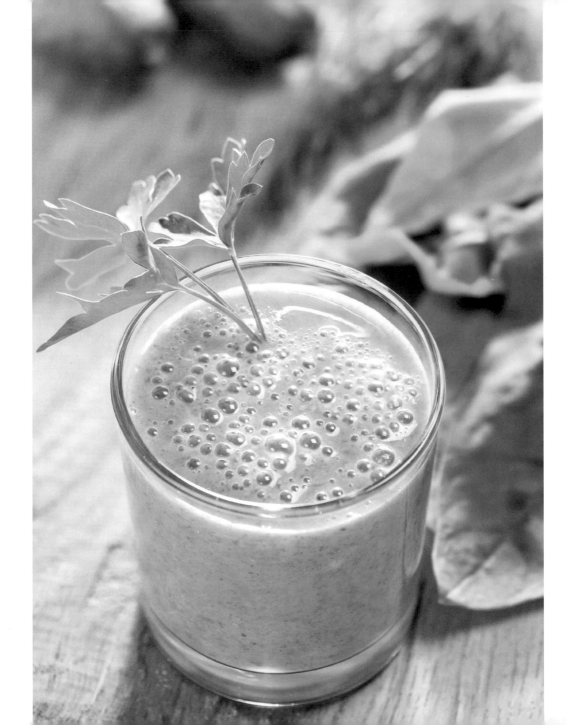

Acknowledgments

I wanted to write this book to make healthy, delicious smoothies accessible to you. Food and nutrition can get complicated, and I prefer it simple. Simple is easy to follow. Simple is easy to integrate into a busy lifestyle. And if simple works, then why not? Smoothies are simple. You don't need to shop at fancy health food stores to make great healthy smoothies. You don't need to get everything organic and locally grown. It would be nice, but it gets expensive and takes longer to plan, and you will have a hard time keeping it up. I want to help you develop a healthy smoothie habit for life by using ingredients found in a typical kitchen and within an average budget.

I feel fortunate that so many wonderful friends, family and fellow smoothie lovers extended their kind support in the writing of this book. First, I want to thank my husband, best friend, and business partner, Andy Brock, for keeping me on task, helping me come up with the best recipes, and going to a smoothie-tasting contest with me to help get all my recipes in order. I want to thank my parents and my husband's parents for being supportive of my vision of helping you return to health and harmony with natural foods. I was thrilled to have the generosity of many companies that sent me samples of their products to test. A complete list of these companies appears after the index. I also want to give a special thanks to all my fabulous recipe contributors: Joshua Waldman, Hollie Jeakins, Rob Cooper, Leslie Broberg, Vickie Velasquez, Adrienne Jurado, Tracy Russell, Jen Hansard, Jadah Sellner, Katherine Natalia, and Jennifer Thompson. They shared their favorite recipes and what led them to healthy smoothies to inspire you to make your own journey to health. Our humble hope is that you will experience it all for yourself. May this book help you find your way back to total health and vitality. Blend away and breathe new life into your body!

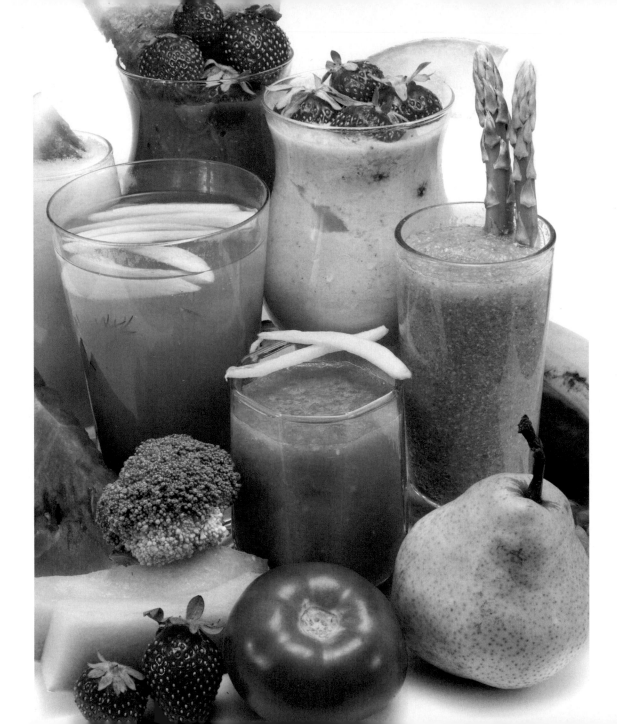

How Best to Use This Book

Are you new to smoothies, or just here for the recipes?

If you are brand-new to smoothies, then please read the book in the right order. I'll introduce you to the smoothie basics, the simple and more complex ingredients (from greens and fruits to nuts and superfoods and other additives), and take you through the preparation and set-up process step by step before we dive into the recipes. Then we talk about cleansing and detoxing with smoothies and easy ways to build smoothies as a sustainable daily habit.

If you are a smoothie pro and are here just for the recipes, then skip over to the Smoothie Recipes section on page 122 for 108 healthy smoothie recipes. You can use the recipes index to find recipes by name or search by major ingredients.

You will also come across a few featured recipes throughout the book from smoothie-lover contributors who have shared their own spin on making a delicious smoothie.

This book can serve as a reference for you over time. As you might know, it's a great idea to rotate your recipes, and especially your greens, so you get a nice variety of ingredients in your system to build up your taste buds as well as get all the vitamins and minerals your body needs. As tempting as it is, don't make the same recipe every day. Not that I can easily convince my own husband when he locks in on his favorite concoctions, but it really is best to switch it up for variety and for maximizing overall nutrition. Plus, variety will keep you intrigued and inspired on your smoothie journey, so don't discount it as you build up your healthy smoothie habit for life.

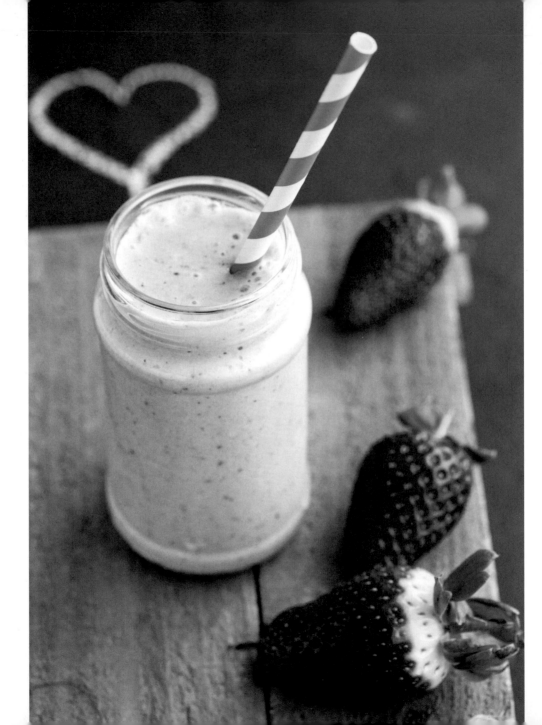

Introduction, and Why Love Is the Path to Smoothies

When diet is wrong, medicine is of no use. When diet is right, medicine is of no need.
~Ayurvedic Proverb

I am in love with the color green in every shade. The green of spinach, kale, Swiss chard, and parsley. The green of lime, cucumber, celery, and green peppers. Simply and utterly in love!

My fascination with green leafy vegetables started in 2007, which I affectionately—albeit seriously—call my "fat year," even though my family and friends still laugh when I refer to it as such, because for reasons that are still beyond my comprehension, none of them will admit to this day that I had grown larger in size, uglier in character, and miserable in spirit that year.

If you want the truth about your health, my advice is not to ask your family or friends. When has anyone in history ever responded truthfully to the question, "Do I look fat?"

We love them and all, but our families and friends always lie about this (although they have good intentions). "Oh, honey, you look great!" comes out automatically, often without really looking at you. Yes, they love you, no matter what, but if your concern is to be your healthiest, happiest, and most energetic, you need to take charge here. It does you no good to be deceived that you are "just fine" when you know that you are far from your optimal health and shape. This is one area of your life in which you need the brutal version of the truth as soon as possible.

Start by looking within yourself for answers: How do you *really* feel about your body? How much *energy* do you really have to get through your days? And how *happy*—or not so happy—are you with yourself and your general state of well-being?

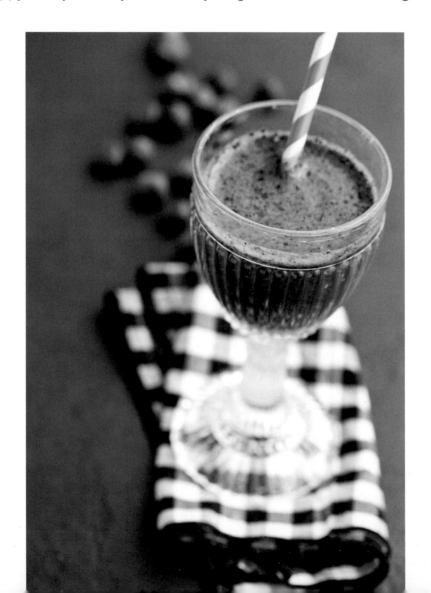

You are your own voice of truth, and it is that voice that will carry you from the depths of any misery, sickness, and sluggishness to better health, more vibrancy, and higher energy. Trust that voice, always!

As for me, when I could no longer deny being miserable in my own body, I started to take baby steps in the right direction.

It was not easy to admit to myself that my health was declining, in part due to my stressful corporate job, which I have long since quit to start my own business. It was no fun to face the fact that I had gained twenty pounds, which was outrageous considering my small frame and my lifelong self-discipline about health and fitness.

Worst of all, it was no picnic to realize that I had been in complete denial about what was happening.

So I started to take action, but this time, I did not follow my usual regimen to getting back in shape, which used to be hitting the gym, ramping up my cardio, and eating less. Those are all wonderful things to do, but I needed a radical change.

I started looking at my nutrition to see if there was a revolutionary way back to health without resorting to fad diets, which I can't stand or follow for the life of me. I needed a permanent shift in lifestyle, one that would be easy enough to sustain *and* delicious and fun enough to make me fall in love. Those were my conditions.

Diets are a temporary solution. What's the point of going on a diet for a while, sticking to a crazy regimen for a few weeks, accomplishing your goals, and then what? Going back to your old ways of eating, and feeling guilty about it to boot?

I'm sorry, but I can't get on board with diets and any kind of strict calorie-counting regimens that only last for a specific period of time. I am not interested in using them for myself or pushing any dietary dogmas or products onto you. Health and vitality is about *feeling great* in your body and your mind, not feeling deprived or restricted just so you reach some goal on the scale.

And feeling great was my measuring stick for returning to health. That is what kept me going down this path of raw foods, green juices, and healthy smoothies. The more I did them, the better, healthier, and happier I felt. They revolutionized my health and well-being, and I want to share my experience and inspire you to do the same for yourself. True health is an everyday endeavor. It's a lifestyle; a way of living that fulfills you, makes you happy, *and* is good to your body.

My journey back to health began with green juicing. That was my first savior. My second godsend, shortly after, was green smoothies. Today, both juices and smoothies fuel my days with a powerhouse of nutrition and energy, as well as the holistic love and care that I had neglected to give my body for a long time.

Juicing and smoothies came into my life as a result of my growing interest in raw and natural whole foods. Confession: I am not, and never have been, a full-time raw foodist, except for a seventeen-day raw vegan challenge in the summer of 2012 and a nine-month vegan period, which I enjoyed immensely. I am also not exclusively on a diet of juices and smoothies. I eat and enjoy solid foods.

But I consume a ton of raw whole foods every day. When I am not on the road, it's a lot easier to keep to my healthy routine. I eat about 60 to 70 percent raw foods during the warmer seasons and about 40 percent during the winter months. When I travel, I look up juice bars and smoothie places. I also take my blender whenever I can, order raw salads, and shop for dark leafy vegetables and fruits in the local grocery stores.

Why the foray into raw foods? I started to study them out of curiosity during my "fat year" in 2007, and I was fascinated by what I learned about the healing and nutritious

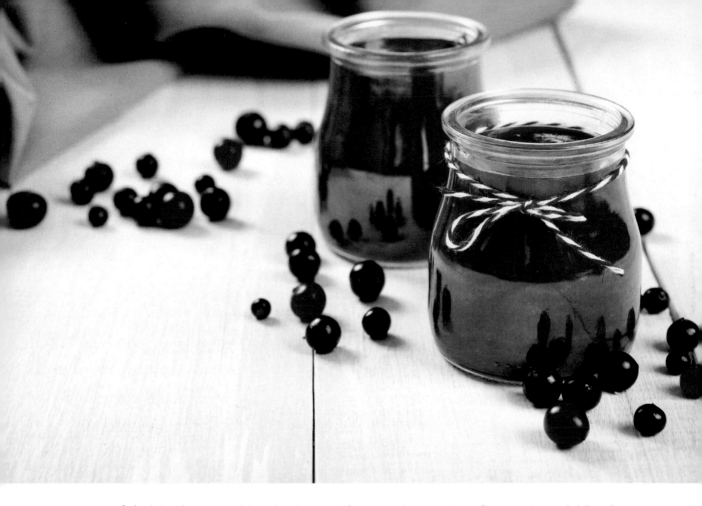

powers of dark leafy vegetables, herbs, and fruits in their various forms—juiced, blended, and whole—and that knowledge sparked my love affair with the world of green (green juices and green smoothies), and years later, I can tell you that the love is stronger every day, and here to stay.

Raw foods, juices, and smoothies have been responsible for not only getting me back on track with my health, but also igniting a deep passion for green juices and green smoothies.

In this book, I share my journey, inspiration, and knowledge about healthy smoothies with you. You will find useful and practical information to get started in the world of delicious smoothies or to kick your current smoothie habit up a notch with 108 delicious recipes and simple ways to create your very own fabulous concoctions.

But more than anything, I want to help you fall madly in love with smoothies.

Inspiration and self-discipline will get you started on this health journey, but to get the real benefit of smoothies, it needs to become a lifestyle and a habit. It needs to turn into your "chocolate craving," and to do that, love is what you need to get there.

You want to build a bond, a tight relationship with your smoothies. You want to make them as much a part of your life as a family member or a beloved pet, and you want to drink your smoothies out of love, not out of obligation.

So on that dreary afternoon when you want a snack and your calendar says, "Drink one large 16-ounce green smoothie," but you just *don't feel like it*? Discipline won't make you do it, and neither will the knowledge about how good it is for you. Instead, your craving for the smoothie taste and that energizing post-smoothie feeling will get you in the mood and excited about making your healthy drink.

Love will drive the smoothie habit and lifestyle for you.

The great news is that smoothies are so within your reach. You don't need to overhaul your entire diet to get started. Just go dust off out your old blender, plug it in, and let's go. Let's dive into the fun and wonderful world of healthy smoothies together. You are here. You are ready. And you are going to fall in love.

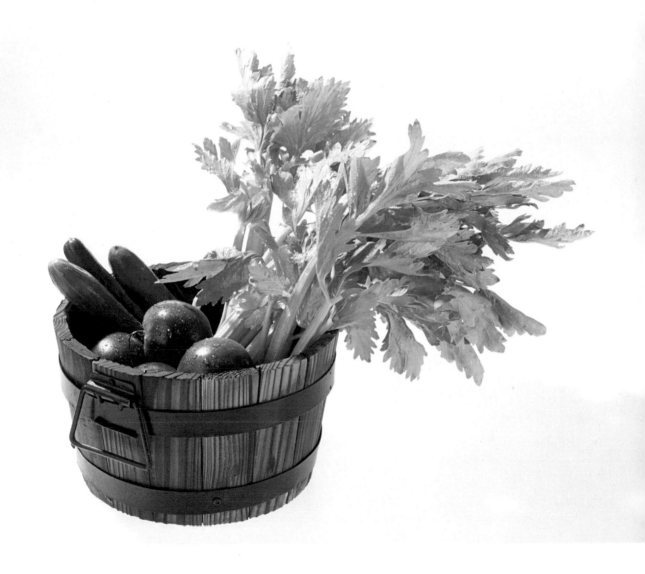

The Healthy Smoothie Magic

If you don't take care of your body, where are you going to live?
~ Unknown

There are many things that can be thrown into the blender and poured into a glass, but just because it looks like a smoothie does not mean it's good for you. It's the same concept as a healthy vegetarian or vegan diet versus a junk vegetarian or vegan diet. Some may argue a junk vegan diet is better than a healthy non-vegan diet. I am not one of them. My mantra is not necessarily to follow an exclusively vegetarian or vegan diet. My mantra is a huge shift in the direction of wholesome, raw, unprocessed, and largely plant-based foods. Healthy smoothies are an extension of that, and done right, they can positively affect your health, your body, and your entire life.

The quick and dirty reason to turn to healthy smoothies is the ease, efficiency, and highly accessible nature of how it works. You need a blender; access to a grocery store or a market that can provide you and your family with fresh fruits, greens, and vegetables; and some know-how, which you are getting by reading this book. That's it! You don't need the complexity of calorie-counting or making special dishes following detailed recipes or finding fancy powders and shakes approved by a brand that claims you will lose X number of pounds while on said diet.

Healthy smoothies are about a shift in your lifestyle that will affect everything from how you feel, look, and approach self-care.

So let's talk about how this happens. What are the benefits, exactly, and what can you expect with a healthy smoothie lifestyle?

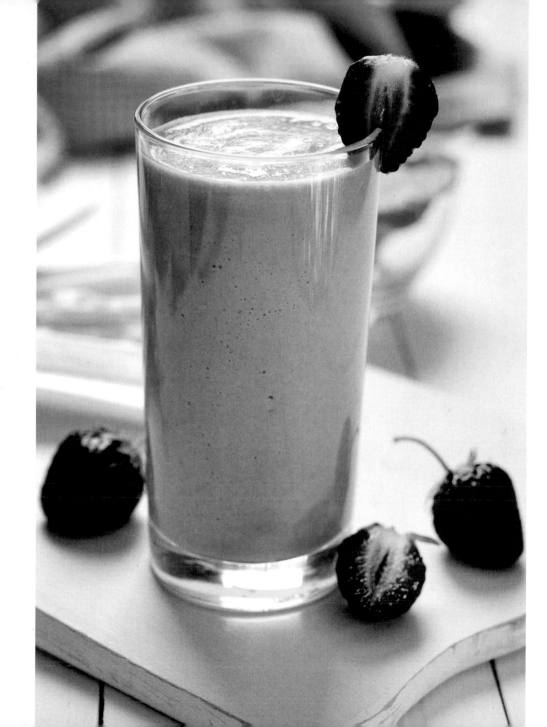

Redefine Your Health, Regain Your Beauty

Health is like money, we never have a true idea of its value until we lose it.
~Josh Billings

Sometimes, one little decision can begin a total transformation.

I remember being paranoid about adding spinach to that first green smoothie. I was standing in the kitchen, holding the spinach with one hand and closing my nostrils with the other, but in they went. The second I smelled that delicious spinach-banana blend, I was hooked! Not only were my taste buds in heaven, my body had found a brand new way to feed itself. Enter smoothies; healthy smoothies and yummy green smoothies.

That little (albeit brave!) decision—adding some spinach into the blender—began my transformation. Let's talk about these green gems so they can become yours.

A *healthy smoothie* is made from a mixture of whole fruits and/or vegetables and sometimes seeds and superfoods, along with a liquid base. You run them through your blender until you achieve a silky smooth texture. You should be able to drink a smoothie with a straw, but if you prefer a thicker consistency, you can also use a spoon. I prefer mine slightly thicker when I am hungrier, and less so when I am looking for hydration. A healthy smoothie does not contain any table sugar, syrups, canned fruit, or artificial sweeteners.

You can make a simple smoothie with just fruits or fruits and vegetables, or go all out and add healthy fats, proteins, and superfoods to turn it into a complete meal. The standard ratio of fruits to vegetables is 60 percent to 40 percent, but you can start with a safer ratio of more fruit first, and add your veggies over time. Over time you may use as much as 80 percent vegetables to 20 percent fruits.

THE HEALTHY SMOOTHIE BIBLE

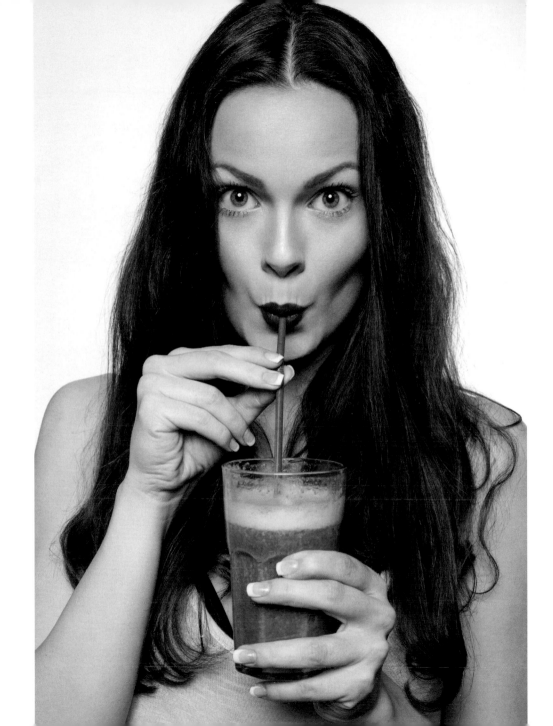

A green smoothie contains a vegetable such as spinach, lettuce, cabbage, parsley, Swiss chard, or any of their cousins. The green smoothie is not so much dictated by its color as it is by what you put into it. Even though you can make some very green-colored smoothies, a few blueberries, blackberries, or one of my favorites, acai powder, can turn the greenest smoothie into a dark purple one. Which can be a nice thing if you are trying to hide the "green factor" for a spouse or a kid, hint hint! The other day I made a cabbage banana smoothie, and it was a beautiful creamy color. That still counts as a green smoothie.

As a general rule, the more green ingredients you use, the higher your smoothie will be on the nutrition scale and the lower on the sugar scale.

By cleansing your body on a regular basis with whole foods and eliminating as many toxins as possible from your diet, your body can begin to heal itself, prevent disease, and become strong and resilient again. No matter how long you have gone down the wrong road, it's not too late to turn it around. Healthy smoothies help you do that in the easiest and fastest way possible. All fruits and vegetables help your body get rid of built-up toxins.

As much as possible, use only organic fresh ingredients in your smoothie recipes, keep it simple with just fruits and vegetables, avoid animal products and artificial sweeteners, and drink your smoothies when they are freshest, which is right after you make them.

Smoothies are the easiest and fastest plunge you can take into natural health and heal-ing. You need very little to get started and equally little time to make them. Your tools of the trade are a decent blender, a cutting board, and a good knife, all of which your average kitchen should already have—plus a little creativity, which this book aims to give you in abundance.

That's it! That's all you need to get going in the art of making a delicious smoothie and revolutionizing your health!

19 Massive Benefits of A Smoothie Lifestyle

A healthy outside starts from the inside.
~Robert Ulrich

I want to emphasize the word "lifestyle" before we talk benefits, because the changes you can enjoy in your health come with building a habit, not after one or two glasses of a smoothie. But you have so much to look forward to once you build the habit, in which you will enjoy three to six smoothies per week. You begin to observe the benefits as early as two weeks in. Here are the top nineteen massive benefits you could get from your healthy smoothie lifestyle:

1. **Makes for a quick and delicious filling snack or meal:** If you are like me, with a busy life and a million things to do, these words are melody to your ears: quick, delicious, filling, and nutritious, all at the same time. A healthy smoothie can give you all of that and more. It can be your breakfast, mid-morning or afternoon snack, or light dinner. You can whip it up and have it ready to go, with everything washed and put away, in less than ten minutes. Now that's a sweet deal!

2. **Provides an excellent source of fiber:** Healthy smoothies are packed with fiber. The fiber is broken down with the power of your blender to where it's easily digestible by your body. Blending your raw, leafy greens not only makes them easier to digest, you also absorb a much higher percentage of nutrients as opposed to chewing them. The fiber lowers your cholesterol and glucose levels, and keeps you fuller longer. Most of all, it regulates your body. This is the biggest benefit of smoothies over juices, which contain little to no fiber.

3. **Makes it easy to get all your nutrients in blended form:** Let's face it. It's a lot of work to prepare and chew your fully recommended dosage of vegetables and fruits.

It takes time to go through all that tonnage. With green smoothies, you drink your greens. You can easily get most of your nutrients into a large glass of a green smoothie before 8:00 a.m.! Now that's efficiency!

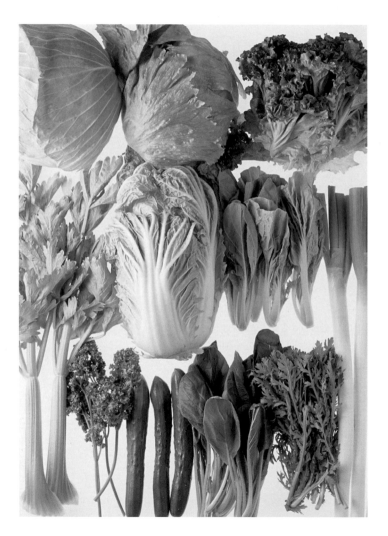

4. **Gives you unlimited flavors (or combinations) to enjoy:** I love fruits and vegetables, I really do, but I do get bored with the singular taste. Even in salads, you still taste individual fruits and vegetables, and I love variety in my mouth! Smoothies open you up to a world of new tastes from the endless combinations you can make. A single fruit or vegetable cannot give you half as much variety on the flavor and fun scale as its blended versions. With a little imagination, you can make countless combinations, and theoretically, you'll never have to make the same exact smoothie twice.

5. **Makes for a portable on-the-go snack:** I remember feeling awkward about taking my container of granola, fruits, and nuts into corporate work meetings. I'd be stealing away a shy little spoonful here and there and not enjoying it at all. With smoothies, they are perfectly portable, easy to suck through a straw, and if anyone gives you a funny look, it's a perfect opportunity to educate them. Seriously, get yourself a nice to-go cup—I like mason jars with glass straws—and make your smoothies to go just as you would any other drink. Just don't drink your smoothie *too* fast. Take sips. Allow it to meet your saliva and then swallow it, rather than chugging it down!

6. **Curbs the cravings for junk food:** I first noticed this when I started switching over to more raw whole foods in my diet, and then with green juicing and smoothies. I used to fight my cravings for bad food with self-discipline and punishment, but it only increased the cravings! The more effective way is to add smoothies to your diet. Over time, you crave more greens and fruits, and after a while, you will not be craving or even tolerating junk foods. What a great cure!

7. **Eases natural weight loss:** Weight loss is no doubt one of the most popular reasons for turning to healthy smoothies, and they work wonders! If you are interested in weight loss, keep your smoothies simple and stick to natural whole foods, monitor the overall calories, use more vegetables and greens, and cut out the nuts, protein powders, and superfoods. Green smoothies especially promote weight loss and melting off those stubborn pounds.

8. **Brings the body to a healthy alkaline state:** The pH balance of human blood needs to stay within a certain range and many foods—especially heavily salted junk foods, fried foods, or packaged foods—are extremely acidic, so your body has to work hard to neutralize their effects and return to its desired state. Fruits and vegetables are alkaline foods, and health experts claim that consuming them helps you maintain a proper alkaline balance in your body. Smoothies help you move in the right direction with your pH balance by acting as a super alkalizer!

9. **Acts as a good source of natural plant proteins:** Believe it or not, plants do have protein. Meat and dairy are not the only sources of protein. Some of the top plant-based protein sources are avocado, broccoli, spinach, and kale, and all of these are yummy ingredients in any smoothie. Smoothies are a great way to consume your plant-based protein, even if you get additional protein from the rest of your diet.

10. **Enhances your digestion and elimination system:** The secret to feeling great is not wealth or riches. It is a great elimination system, and you would agree if you have ever been deprived of yours for even a little while. Constipation and indigestion are no fun, and that alone can be your greatest incentive to start a healthy smoothie habit. The fiber in the fruits and vegetables and the easy absorption of those fibers helps you regulate yourself and create a robust system to withstand a wonderfully long and productive life.

11. **Boosts your energy and vitality:** Smoothies are a smart way to fuel your body before a workout or to recover after a workout. They can give you a boost of energy without weighing you down, as most recommended post-workout, heavy, protein-rich meals tend to do. You get a natural boost of energy and a feeling of invigoration and hydration at the same time, thanks to all the fresh raw fruits and vegetables in your smoothie. Where was this genius meal when I needed it after my aerobic classes as a teenager?

12. **Increases your immune system against colds and illness:** Whole foods are a miracle for your immune system, and healthy smoothies do their part in increasing your body's ability to resist and fight infections. The healthier your body, the quicker you can fight off the onset of a cold or illness. Increase your green smoothies when you feel weak or fatigued to expedite the healing or do away with the whole cold or flu before it sets in.

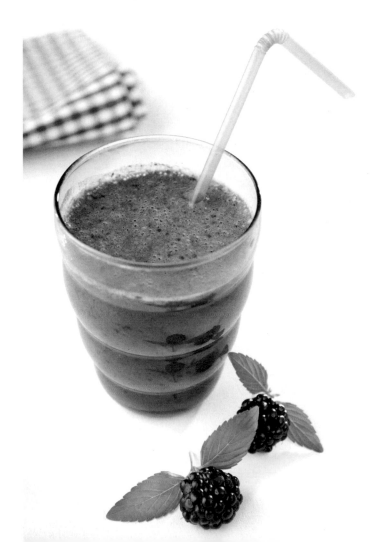

13. **Gives your skin a glow and your hair a shine:** Real beauty is on the inside, I agree, but can we also care about the outer beauty? Your skin, your nails, your hair are going to love the shine and glow that you get from a regular healthy smoothie habit. Your body's outer beauty is a function of how well it is doing on the inside, and smoothies do a great job on that inside. So good, you'll be glowing soon.

14. **Saves money in the long run:** Smoothies are very budget-friendly. You can freeze your fruits so none goes to waste, pick vegetables that are in season, and shop at your farmer's markets to buy in bulk. Plus you can keep your recipes simple without the froo-froo of all the superfoods and exotic herbs. And here's the hidden bonus: smoothies improve your health, and you also save money by not running to the doctor or drug-store as frequently.

15. **Easily accommodates all diet types:** You're vegan? Raw? Gluten-free? Allergic to nuts? Avoiding soy? High on greens? Going slow-carb or low-carb? Whatever your nutritional needs and desires, smoothies are extremely open to modification. You can whip up delicious recipes for your exact needs and have plenty of variety while sticking to your dietary choices.

16. **Teaches you about natural healing with the right foods:** Smoothies are a great, fun way to get curious and learn about healing your body with food, not medicine. A lot of our physical ailments and aches and pains can be traced back to poor nutrition, but the good news is you can heal most of them and feel better by consciously choosing the right foods for your body. You can experiment to your heart's content by bringing the healing from fruits and vegetables and herbs into a glass of smoothie.

17. **Gives you an effortless way to eat more raw foods:** Raw foods are the staple of a healthy diet, and even though I'm not 100 percent raw, I enjoy a lot of raw foods in my diet. But it's a challenge to get creative with raw foods, and it takes a lot of energy to chew all the raw foods that you need. Smoothies are a magical way to help you get your raw foods with little effort.

18. **Allows your creativity to shine:** I am not a cook, and I can't bake for the life of me, but I fell in love with juicing and smoothies because they let me get creative without burning the kitchen down or causing any other unmitigated disasters that you have to worry about as a chef. With smoothies, you get to explore the world of fruits, vegetables, herbs, nuts, and seeds, and it's a big wide world. A fabulous outlet for a "zen" kind of creativity.

19. **Makes you happy:** This one you won't believe until you do it, but after you have whipped up a few delicious concoctions of your own, you will notice the joy and happiness a glass of smoothie can bring. Our bodies crave good nutrition and delicious taste, a combination that we have to remember to nurture it with, and the natural reaction of your body is happiness. I still get a giggle from my concoctions, and a smile so big that I forget my troubles for a few minutes a day! Life is good already, but it's so much better with smoothies.

The number of benefits from healthy smoothies is so long that I can't possibly cover every amazing physical, mental, psychological, and emotional goodness that will result from drinking your healthy smoothies regularly. This is just the beginning of an exciting and delicious journey, and you won't look back once you start.

Smoothies versus Juices: Which is Better?

You are as important to your health as it is to you.
~Terri Guillemets

You may hear people interchange the words *juicing* and *smoothies*, but they are not the same thing. In short: with juicing, you extract the fiber and drink just the juice, and you typically need a juicer to do this. With smoothies, you blend everything and drink the result, fiber and all.

Some find that juicing is more wasteful, with all that pulp that you don't drink. True, but you can repurpose that pulp in many ways. Juicing can also be more expensive; it yields less per pound or kilogram of fruits and vegetables than a smoothie because all of the pulp is extracted. Nothing is lost in the blending process of a smoothie, except for the change in the physical volume of food that goes from solid to liquid form.

One compelling reason people choose juicing is because of its fasting benefits. You can fast on juices and give your digestive system a rest and your body a reboot, if you will. By the same token, people gravitate towards smoothies because they like to get fiber in their diets. A juicer will extract the fiber so that you are only getting the juice, whereas a Vitamix or a similarly powerful blender will break down the fiber considerably, and you are drinking the whole thing. Smoothies are food—complete foods that can fill you up and keep you happy a good few hours—whereas juices are absorbed faster, give you a quicker energy boost, and are less filling in comparison. However, there is still a way to modify your smoothies in order to do a Detox & Cleanse, which we cover on page 211.

So which approach should you take? I suggest both! They are both very good for you. I love both juices and smoothies. They're both like my children. Just as you'd never ask a mother to choose between her children, I'd never give up one over the other.

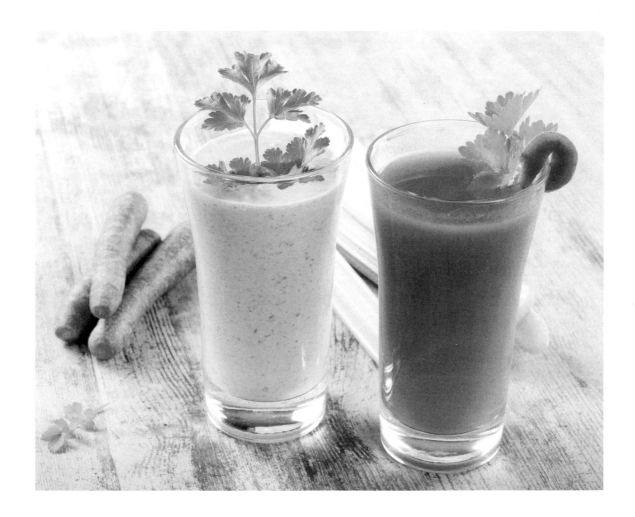

Now, here are the guidelines to help you decide whether to blend or to juice:

Both juicing and blending are fantastic for you. Juice if it suits your fancy, or whip up a smoothie if you are in the mood for one. Do one or the other or *both*. Don't get too

Blend if:
- You want a filling meal to keep you satisfied for a few hours.
- You are in a hurry and need to do it fast.
- You want the fiber in your fruits and vegetables.
- You want to use fruits such as banana and avocado that do not juice.
- You want to toss in your supplements, seeds, powders, and other superfoods.
- You have both the appetite and time to consume a smoothie.
- You are more hungry than thirsty.

Juice if:
- You want to quickly absorb the minerals and vitamins in the vegetables and fruits.
- You want to consume a large variety and volume of fruits and vegetables fast.
- You want a flood of nutrition without any of the fiber.
- You want a hydrating drink.
- You want to rest your digestive system for a few hours or for longer.
- You want to detox and cleanse your system without fiber.
- You want a quick energy boost.
- You are more thirsty and dehydrated than hungry.

caught up in the fuss and heated polarized debates between the juice camps and the smoothie camps. I highly recommend that you incorporate both juices and smoothies into your diet if you can. The main downside of doing both is that you would need two separate machines, both a juicer and a blender. I've made that investment into my health and don't regret it at all. I hope you make the right decision for you, now that you better understand the difference between juicing and blending.

My recommendation is to avoid bottled juices and bottled smoothies unless the label specifically says cold-pressed, never heated, and that the drink contains no additional chemicals or processed sugars. Most bottled health drinks have been pasteurized, which diminishes the nutrient potency and alters the taste. You wouldn't even recognize the taste if you were to make a fresh version of what you get from such a bottle!

I also recommend you pass up on chain smoothie shops. They usually just have limited fruit options for smoothies and tend to add extra artificial sweeteners on top. I long to see a day when the smoothie shops stock up on spinach and kale next to the berry section, but it may be a while. Leafy vegetables perish quickly, whereas you can keep frozen fruit much longer. Some health food stores, such as select Whole Foods locations, have a setup that allows you to shop from their produce section and have it directly made into a smoothie or juice at their juice bar. Now that's awesome, and worth doing at least once! Big cities might even surprise you with their fresh vegan raw food movements. I have enjoyed green smoothies in Toronto, Canada, in the underground shops, Portland's many vegan stops, as well as Hawaii's well-hidden raw vegan cafes, but they are still an uncommon sight. Your best option is to make your own healthy green smoothie and juice concoctions at home.

The most important takeaway is this: Drink Your Greens. Be it green juice, green smoothie, or a mix, drinking your greens will move you closer to a more healthy, vibrant version of you.

No juicing is necessary to create your smoothies. I have certainly made recipes that required fresh carrot or orange juice to be mixed in with the smoothie ingredients. But since I would rather you skip juices in bottled form, and since I would not want you to have to clean two machines—a juicer and a blender—just to make a smoothie, we have no fresh juice requirement in any of the recipes in this book. The only thing I ask you to do is to squeeze the juice of a lemon or a lime into the blender on some occasions, and that you can do with your bare hands.

You can check out my last book, *The Healthy Juicer's Bible*, to learn more about juicing. Now let's focus on how you can make healthy smoothies a part of your diet and lifestyle.

Joshua Waldman

Favorite Recipe: Tropical Pineapple Dream

½ fresh pineapple
1 peeled orange
⅛ lime, unpeeled
1–2 handfuls fresh spinach
2–3 ice cubes
1 cup filtered water

Joshua likes to slice a one-centimeter sliver all the way across the lime and throw it in. After he puts the fruit in, he fills the rest of the blender up with spinach, maybe one or two handfuls, then adds six ice cubes or one cup of water, or a mix of the two, and blends away. It turns florescent green and is super yummy. It fills you up and gives your body lots of phytonutrients.

Joshua Waldman is an authority on leveraging social media to find employment. He is the author of *Job Searching With Social Media For Dummies* and runs a popular career blog at CareerEnlightenment.com. When he's not writing, Joshua presents keynotes, trainings around the world for students, career advisors, and professional organizations. Joshua is also a lover of whole foods, raw juices, and green smoothies. He grows his own herbs and wheatgrass at home, and he relies on the power of holistic nutrition for keeping him sharp, healthy, and active. He dedicates this smoothie to his wife, Lily.

Why Dairy-Free Smoothies?

If you desire healing, let yourself fall ill, let yourself fall ill.
~Rumi

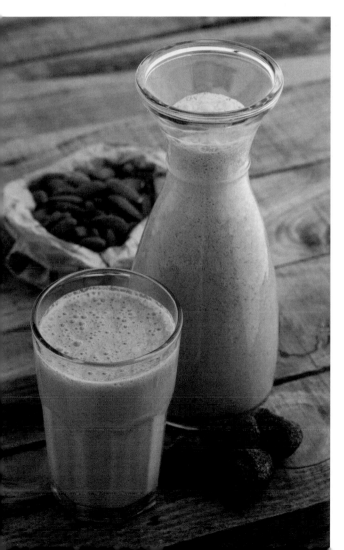

All of my smoothie recipes in this book are dairy-free. You may find dairy in some of the contributed recipes that are featured at the end of each chapter. I personally do not use any animal milk or yogurt products in my smoothies. I have lactose intolerance, plus just a personal vendetta against animal milk—sorry, milk lovers! And while I enjoy plain yogurt on rare occasions by itself—I'm from Iran, and I grew up eating plain yogurt as a mandatory part of our Persian feasts—I still do not mix any yogurt into my healthy smoothies. You have so many better options for making your smoothies nice and creamy without adding the dairy in, and that's the smoothie journey I hope to get you excited about.

If you are worried about getting your calcium, relax. You can get plenty of calcium from leafy green vegetables and nuts without any dairy. Milk and yogurt contain excess fat, sugar, hormones, and other additives that sabotage your goals to get healthy, detox your body, or lose weight. Use dark leafy greens and fruits such as oranges, kiwi, figs, pears, and dates to get your calcium.

Also, when you use fortified nut milks from brands such as Silk, Blue Diamond, and Rice Dreams, you enjoy the added calcium, as well as the vitamin D your body needs to absorb the calcium. Nut milks do not contain any lactose, which is the acidic stuff in cow's milk to which many of us have a huge sensitivity or plain intolerance. And last but not least, if you have not tasted nut milks until now, your taste buds are in for a treat!

I also do not use or advocate soy milk. Soy products tend to be allergenic foods, and most soy is filled with phytoestrogens, so it could negatively affect your hormonal balance. All in all, it is not a choice of base that I recommend, but you can certainly use it if you like the taste. Recent studies about nutrition do not favor using a lot of soy in your diet. You get far better nutrition and taste by using nut milks as your base. My all-time favorites are unsweetened almond milk, unsweetened coconut milk, or a combination of the two. I've tried rice milk, as well as hemp milk, but rice milk is bland, and I prefer hemp seeds to the hemp milk.

As you can see, you have lots of options with non-dairy milks and can use your favorite in all the non-water-based recipes.

If you feel strongly about having some milk or yogurt in your smoothie, by all means, feel free to add it. Remember, you are in charge. This is your smoothie, and it has to work for your taste buds. Yogurt is popular as a smoothie base and is known to add a nice consistency to smoothies, but frankly, you can get a similar or even a better consistency with bananas, avocados, and nut butters. Just sayin'!

This book gives you suggestions and ideas. I hope that you will give the dairy-free smoothie an honest try. That's what the smoothie journey is all about: to expand beyond your comfort zone, and to play and find combinations of fruits and vegetables and other nutrients that are devilishly delicious. You can't find those combinations if you only stick to what you know. I've done the homework here so you don't have to go figuring it all out. All you have to do is be willing to try the recipes. You might just be pleasantly surprised!

The recipes here contain any combination of frozen or fresh fruits, fresh vegetables, fresh herbs, seeds, nut milks (almond, coconut) or rice milk or filtered water base, and nut butters, as well as dairy-free protein powders and select superfoods. Always modify according to your own needs and preferences.

The War on Fructose: Does Fruit Make You Fat?

Happiness lies, first of all, in health.
~George William Curtis

Fruit. One of the healthiest, most delicious, and most naturally occurring foods on the planet. We eat it to satiate our hunger, our thirst, and our taste buds, all at the same time. Man (and woman) have been eating fruit for millennia, or even longer, for all we know.

Fruit is good for you.

Fruit does not make you fat. Do you know anyone who has gotten fat from eating too much ripe, fresh, whole fruit? Do you really believe that America's obesity epidemic is caused by eating too much fruit? It's the obsession with processed sugar and junk food that has caused the epidemic. I would challenge you to gain any weight by eating only fruit all day long. It just won't happen.

When you look at the food consumption on the average American diet, you will see a sad dearth of fruit (among other things), and yet we have a large and growing epidemic of diseases that are a result of the Standard American Diet (SAD) and still find time to blame fruit for "causing sugar spikes" and tossing it aside as high carb and therefore "bad for you."

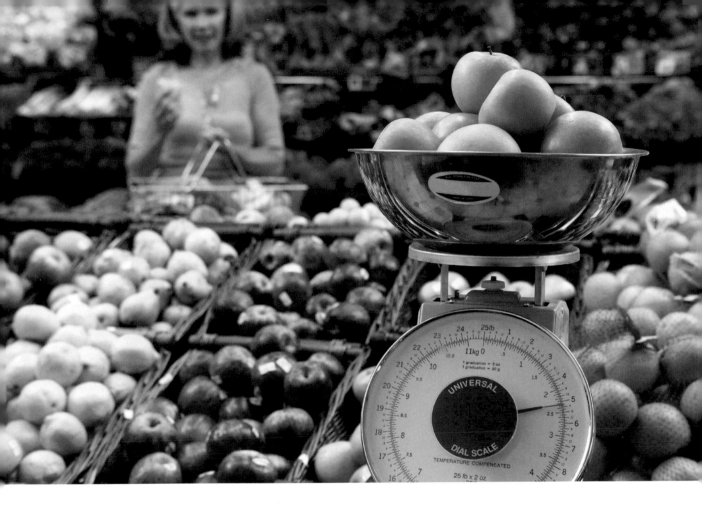

Fruit is not bad for you. Kill that thought now! The sugar in fruit is not the same sugar as in doughnuts, cookies, cakes, and candy. There is no argument that the refined sugars in those types of foods are bad for you. Really bad for you. Those are definitely in the bad carbohydrate category. Fruit is not in the same category. But if you have been eating a diet high in sugar and poor in nutrition, then adding fruit on top of that is not a good idea.

With healthy smoothies, you will begin your return to healthy eating, and your body will be cleansing and healing from the effects of poor nutrition. If that's you, then you may want to consider greener smoothies lower in sugar (look for the right recipe tags to identify these) and as you build up your health, then you can easily add fruit to your smoothies and to the rest of your diet as whole foods on their own.

The naturally occurring sugar in fruit is known as fructose, but that's not the only thing found in fruit. Fruit also contains fiber, which helps slow down the breakdown of said sugar into your bloodstream, as opposed to all the junk food, which instantly gets into your bloodstream. It is critical to eat your fruits and use at least some fruit as a foundation in your smoothies. Fruit has a relatively low glycemic index, and you would have to consume enormous amounts of it to be of any potential harm. A sixteen- or twenty-ounce smoothie per day containing some fruit will not be able to do that kind of harm! Also, adding leafy vegetables, nuts, and seeds to your smoothie balances out the overall sugar.

But here's the thing. Fruit also contains lots of vitamins, minerals, and antioxidants, including Vitamin C, potassium, and, of course, the aforementioned fiber that counterbalances any potential harm you could possibly get from its natural sugars. Fruit makes your skin glow, aids with both weight-loss and digestion, and is one of the staples of a healthy, raw-friendly diet.

Please note that if you are diabetic or have diabetic tendencies or any other metabolic diseases, I highly recommend you discuss this with your doctor.

All the same, I respect that you may not wish to have much or any fruit in your smoothie, so I have included several recipes that provide low-carb options with little to no fruit added. Check for the smart recipe tag "Low Fruit" to locate these recipes.

Smoothies as Meal Replacement or Just a Snack?

Healing comes from taking responsibility: to realize that it is you—and no one else—that creates your thoughts, your feelings, and your actions.
~Peter Shepherd

You can make smoothies for meal replacement or just as a snack. When you are starting out, the idea of replacing a whole meal with a drink may be intimidating,

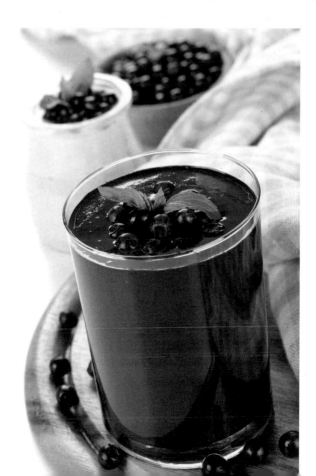

so don't worry about it ahead of time. Just add smoothies to your regular diet and let the rest take care of itself. For example, have your smoothie for breakfast, and eat your regular meal or regular "breakfast" afterwards *only* if you are hungry. You will soon realize that smoothies can be quite filling and satisfying, and it's not difficult to replace them for an entire meal and go a few hours without needing to snack.

If you are trying to lose some weight with smoothies, then start by replacing one meal a day with a green smoothie and then work up to two smoothies a day with a light dinner. This can be a great way to kick-start your weight loss plan.

Here are some tips on how to make a snack smoothie versus a meal replacement smoothie.

A Meal Replacement Smoothie:

A meal replacement smoothie should have between 400 to 600 calories. The idea of a meal replacement is to fill you up, give you lots of nutrition, and satiate your body so you are not hungry an hour or so later. When I make my meal replacement smoothies, I usually like to add fruits and vegetables (those are the staples), some nuts or nut butters, and either some brown rice protein powder or a source of omega-3 fatty acids like hemp seeds or chia seeds. I also tend to use nut milk as base instead of just water, but it does depend on the recipe. These smoothies are generally thicker and more substantial than a snack smoothie. I drink anywhere between twenty and thirty ounces without an ounce of guilt!

If I'm not ready to drink all of it at once, I have a two-part meal and drink half of it right after I make it, then store the other half in the refrigerator in a glass container with a tight lid. Then I clean up the blender, make some hot oolong tea to help digest my "first meal," and an hour later, I would have part two of my meal. This helps me avoid the super-full feeling that can weigh you down simply from having a large drink. The difference with smoothies as opposed to, say, a feast of Indian food, is that you will soon digest your smoothie and most of the water weight will leave your body through urine. The Indian meal, on the other hand, can keep your belly heavy for an entire afternoon!

A Snack Smoothie:

If you want to have a smoothie just as a snack, make a smaller serving and opt for a more hydrating option than a filling one. Check out the water-based recipes in this book, and use half the portions to make yourself a snack serving. Also avoid putting nut butters and protein powders in a snack smoothie, so you can keep the fat content down. Keep it heavy on fruits and vegetables, but go light on the heavier fruits like avocado and banana.

I like a snack smoothie when I am not quite hungry enough for a meal. Mid-afternoon can be a great time to make a snack smoothie, or you can make it earlier in the day and store it for a few hours to have it ready to go. If you have the luxury of making it fresh, do! You can also go with your cravings and make the right fruits and veggies that you are in the mood for.

Hollie Jeakins

Favorite Recipe: Chocolate Mango "Ice Cream" Smoothie Delight

¾ cup coconut milk
1 cup frozen mango chunks
1 tbsp cacao or cocoa
½ tsp chia seeds
¼ tsp coconut oil (optional)

Place ingredients listed into blender (starting with coconut milk) and process on high until smooth and creamy. Enjoy this "ice cream" smoothie as a super clean after-dinner indulgence. The sweet mango, raw cacao, and creamy coconut milk combine to create the perfect end to a delicious meal.

Hollie shares step-by-step articles, mouthwatering recipes, and healthy eating inspiration with thousands of loyal readers through her popular blog, SimplyWholeFoods.com. Her focus is on soy-free, gluten-free and paleo-friendly recipes that are perfectly suited for those with allergies and intolerances, or those who just want to make healthy choices for themselves and their families. Hollie lives near Toronto, Canada, with her beloved husband and her two precious children. The smoothie would be good anytime, but you could definitely include it in a healthy dessert smoothie category!

Ingredients 101 for the Perfect Smoothie

If we are what we eat and we don't know what we are eating, then do we still know who we are?
~Claude Fiscler

What goes into your healthy smoothie is just as important as what stays out of it! Let's talk ingredients, freshness, combinations, liquid base, guidelines on mixing and matching, and what not to put in your smoothie. It's easy to have the best of intentions and then kill a great smoothie with a shot of syrup (something you should never put in your smoothie). The easiest way to approach your smoothie is to use fresh raw green leafy vegetables, combined with fresh or frozen fruit and some filtered water. With that basic foundation, you can figure out whatever combination your heart desires, and the result will be a healthy smoothie because your ingredients are raw, fresh, and preferably with a shade or two of green.

Not all healthy smoothies have greens in them or come out green in color. If you choose to only make a smoothie with fruits and some water, that works. Yes, it may be sweeter than a green smoothie, but it is still healthy fruit in blended form with plenty of fiber to allow for the slower release of fructose into your blood cells. It beats a cookie, a bag of chips, or a slice of cake any day of the week. Greens just up the scale of nutrients and minerals, as well as balance out the sweetness of a fruit-only smoothie. We will talk about how to get over your fear of adding greens into a perfectly fine fruit smoothie, and which greens and fruits to seek out.

Beyond the fresh produce, you can get a little fancy with superfoods, seeds, and protein powders. I've included my experience here, and the main takeaway is this: Your (green) healthy smoothie is your superfood, but you can get an even higher boost of

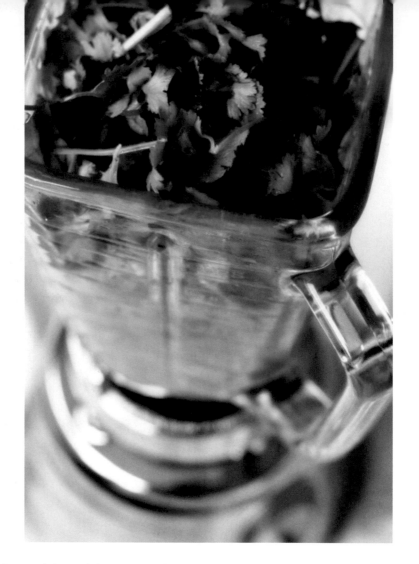

nutrition, if desired, by adding something extra. This is not necessary; it is a "would-be-nice" feature.

Soon you will be mixing and matching your favorite flavors and becoming a master of smoothie ingredients. Let's get started down the discovery path!

The Scoop on the Greens for Your Smoothies

There is more evidence than ever before that dietary choices have major impacts on population health.
~Food & Drug Administration

How to Get Over Your Fear of Mixing Greens in Your Smoothie

If you are like me and many others, you'll feel a wee bit of paranoia the first time you want to add a handful of spinach to a perfectly good fruit smoothie, and that fear is not without good reason. For starters, I don't know of any culture where traditional meals are served with a mixed blend of fruits and vegetables, especially in the color green. Do you? Salads are every culture's claim to "healthy" food, but salads are considered to be a *side dish*. A little iceberg lettuce (zero nutrition, mainly water), along with a few random vegetables and topped with a highly fattening dressing is not exactly going to warm you up to your greens!

And your goal is not just to warm up to your greens, but to *fall in love* with them!

So my best tip for getting over your fear of mixing greens into your smoothie is this: Take a big leap of faith and know that you have nothing to lose (and everything to gain)!

Think of it this way. You already know what greens taste like, and you know what fruits taste like, but what you may not know is that blending them gives you a brand-new taste. It's not the green taste, which may be bland or bitter to your taste buds, and it's not the sweet fruit taste. It is however, positively heavenly. I am not a chemist, so I can't give you a scientific answer, but I'll have to ask you to trust me on this one. Green smoothies are a new taste altogether!

Plus, variety is the spice of life, and one of the reasons I LOVE green smoothies is because I can create a new concoction and therefore a new taste without much effort, and my taste buds never have to grow bored.

So, now that you're ready to go for it, start with the "Hidden Greens" tagged recipes, and see for yourself. Green smoothies are going to revolutionize the way you see, think, and even dream about your greens. The idea behind this tag is to slowly ease a beginner—you or someone in your family—into green smoothies before they get to the more advanced recipes.

SMOOTHIE LOVER IN THE SPOTLIGHT

Rob Cooper

Favorite Recipe: The Blended Salad Smoothie

1–2 handfuls of mixed greens
1 celery stalk
1–2 leaves of kale
2–4 inches of cucumber, unpeeled
1 handful parsley
1–2 medium carrots
1–2 oz of your favorite nut (almonds, walnuts, or cashews)
Optional: Chia seeds, hemp hearts

Rob mixes this recipe up with different greens, such as organic baby lettuces (red and green romaine, red and green oak leaf, red leaf, lollo rosa, tango), organic mizuna, organic red and green chard, organic baby spinach, organic arugula,

---

organic frisee, organic radicchio. He buys the one-pound clamshell containers of organic spring mix from his local grocer when out of season in the yard. Carrots, cucumber, and celery provide the liquid base, so no need to add extra water. Consider that when choosing your numbers for the items. Parsley can dramatically affect the flavor, Rob says, so choose an amount based on your preference for the flavor, offset by the high nutritional value of the plant. Add avocado for a creamy texture.

The blended salad is to be a full-bodied savory meal, as he doesn't like them sweet. You may add some apple for some sweetness. He doesn't usually like combining fruits with any other foods, but apple and raspberry work all right if you decide to add them. No salad dressings should be added. Blended salads provide a whole food supplement, including naturally distilled plant water, vitamins, minerals, fat, chlorophyll, and more in a pre-digested meal or side dish. They contain all the original fiber while at the same time providing slow-release nutrient delivery with lower impact on blood sugar. Fast food for Rob is a BBQ steak or salmon with his blended salad. Little or no dishes to do afterward and he takes his "salad" drink everywhere he goes.

Once weighing 475 pounds, Rob Cooper is now living a lifestyle of health in Western Canada. He has run the popular blog and website, FormerFatGuy.com, since 2000 and is the author of *Fat Loss Fundamentals*. He's fascinated by the subject of change and loves studying gardening, permaculture, and sustainable living. He swings kettlebells and sources out pasture-raised, grass-fed beef, pork, chicken, and eggs. He eats a paleo diet.

Which Greens to Use in Your Smoothies?

My go-to favorites are spinach, lettuce, parsley, and kale in the dark leafy veggies category, but that's just the beginning. You have lots and lots of options. Start with your favorite ones on the list and rotate them.

This is a great time to get curious and interested in learning about greens. What's in season? What's bitter versus mild? What's bland versus tangy? What has aroma or spice? The more you learn about your greens, the more you can take charge of your smoothie journey.

As much as possible, I recommend getting your greens in the organic produce section and using them at their freshest. This is one of the big challenges of green smoothies, because vegetables tend to perish faster than fruits. Check out my shopping and prepping tips to make your greens last longer. If you are watching your budget, organic can get expensive, but if nothing else, strive to purchase organic leafy greens.

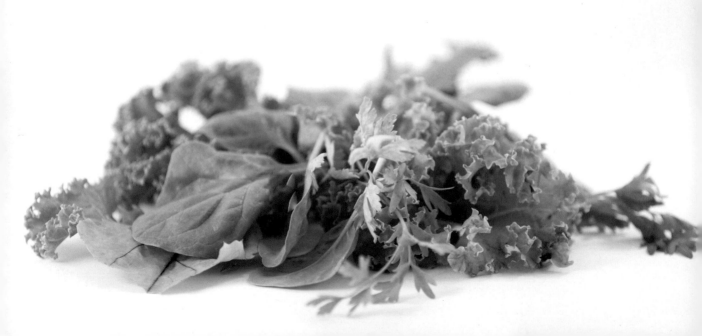

Why You Should Rotate Your Greens

It's important to rotate your greens. Here are two reasons for doing this:

1. **Nutritional diversity:** You want to get as many nutrients as possible, so using the same old spinach or parsley for every green smoothie won't cover all your bases. When you rotate your greens, you get a wider range of minerals and nutrients in different greens.

2. **Potential toxic avoidance:** There is a tiny level of toxins in each green, and it's usually a different kind in each one. Eating two or three servings a day is fine, but in order to avoid a build-up of these chemicals in your body over time, avoid using the same exact green for weeks at a time.

An easy way to do this is either to add variety every time you make a smoothie, or to tell yourself that you'll have, say, spinach and parsley for say two weeks, then switch it up to kale and mint for the next two weeks, and lettuce and cilantro after that before you resume spinach again. Ideally you want to switch up between different plant families, as the same plant family picks up the same toxin traces.

You do not need to rotate your fruits as long as you avoid eating the seeds. But to get full nutritional diversity, you should be mixing it up in the fruit section too.

You know what this means right? Your fun challenge now is to learn about all the beautiful vegetables and fruits in your produce section or at your farmer's market. Don't get stuck in a rut! Rotate, explore, and have fun!

Remember to always use fresh greens in your smoothies. Never use frozen greens! The easy way to remember is this: If it has leaves, don't freeze it. Most fruits and some vegetables, like avocado, can be frozen (a later section on this), but never freeze your greens!

The Top Ten Greens of Choice for Your Smoothie

I have not by any measure listed ALL the greens you could be using in your smoothies. These are the top ten that I rotate through frequently and have used in the recipes. There are many others. Feel free to explore any green you like. Always start in small quantities—a fraction of a handful—and taste the green by itself to judge the level of bitterness before tossing it in.

Here are the top ten greens of choice that I recommend starting with. Greens are a subset of vegetables that are mainly dark and leafy and lightweight. The list is in no particular order:

Spinach: Spinach is the one green that you will hardly ever taste in your smoothie. It is the ultimate starter green if you are new to smoothies. It is also one of the most nutrient-rich leafy greens. It is easy to find spinach in just about any store, it's pretty affordable, and full of minerals and phytonutrients. It's an excellent source of vitamin K, vitamin A, magnesium, folate, manganese, iron, calcium, vitamin C, vitamin B2, potassium, and vitamin B6. Spinach is also a very good source of protein, phosphorus, vitamin E, zinc, dietary fiber, and copper.

Kale: Kale is a little harder to find, but it's becoming more popular. It lasts longer than spinach in the fridge because of its thicker texture. It comes in several different types, and all are perfectly fine for smoothies. You can take off the stem to remove some of the bitterness. Kale is stronger than spinach but not bitter, per se. Kale is low in calories; high in iron and vitamin K, vitamin A, and calcium; and filled with antioxidants. Incorporate this in your smoothies over time.

Parsley: Parsley is a beautiful herb; it can have a strong yet flavorful taste, but it's also perfect for reducing sweetness in a smoothie if need be, and it works with all fruits and veggies. Parsley is a great source of folic acid, an important B vitamin that your body needs. Similar to kale, it's a great source of vitamins A, C, and K, as well as iron. Parsley is not a garnish. Eat your parsley or throw a handful in your smoothie to make it super green and super healthy.

Cilantro: You either love or hate cilantro. I happen to love it. If you haven't had it, taste it before using it in your smoothies. Cilantro is a great herb that opens up the flavor of food, and it can add a nice taste to your smoothies. Use just a small handful if you choose it as an ingredient. Cilantro is rich in magnesium, iron, and phytonutrients; helps reduce blood sugar; and is a very healing herb.

Swiss chard: This is a colorful leafy green with thicker skin than spinach, and it has a distinct taste. It will last longer than spinach in the fridge, and it adds rich red and green colors to your smoothie. It is a powerhouse of nutrients similar to all its cousins here, rich in vitamins A, C, and K, as well as a source of potassium, iron, and magnesium. Taste it before using in your smoothie. It goes a long way, and you can start with just one stalk.

Lettuce: Try not to use iceberg lettuce, as it is void of any nutrition. Romaine lettuce is the best and most nutritious type of lettuce, and it blends beautifully in your smoothies. You can also explore other types of lettuce, such as Boston lettuce, red or green leaf lettuce, or escarole. All the lettuce recipes in this book use romaine lettuce. Romaine has vitamins C and K and is brilliant for weight loss, as well as being a great source of potassium.

Dandelion: These leafy greens are strong and bitter, so adopt them slowly into your routine. They are there if you want to kick things up a notch. Dandelions have spinach beat with their iron content (but spinach wins on the vitamin C and folate scales!), plus they are a great source of vitamin A, E (not common in all greens), and K. Including a couple of dandelion leaves sparingly will add some kick to your smoothies and help you rotate those greens. Again, start with small doses until you're comfortable with their taste.

Collard greens: With their thick skin and large leaves, these are pretty giant to buy and store, but so good for you. Collard greens have a milder taste than kale, and they have similar levels of vitamin A, vitamin C, vitamin K, iron, folate, and magnesium as the other greens listed here. Even though these greens are not as sexy and adored as spinach and kale, they are a powerhouse of nutrition, and it's best to include them in your greens rotation.

Basil: A highly fragrant herb, it can add flavor and aroma to your smoothies, plus it has its fair share of antioxidants and a good source of Vitamin K. It also helps with digestion and can be good for your skin. It is an expensive herb, so use it whenever you have access to it.

Mint: Also a highly fragrant herb, mint is a lovely addition to your smoothies. Mint's best known for helping with indigestion, and it gives you good breath. Mint is also rich in manganese, vitamin A, and vitamin C. It also is a good source of fiber, folate, iron, vitamin B2, potassium, and copper, and it is delicious. You already know the taste of mint, so using it in your smoothies should be fun and easy.

Carrot tops: Did you know carrots actually have green tops? You don't always see them in the store, but if you shop at your farmer's market, that's how they sell carrots. You'll want to save and use those beautiful long carrot tops as a green for your smoothies. They are strong and somewhat bitter, but highly nutritious, and even one or two stalks are enough to get you started.

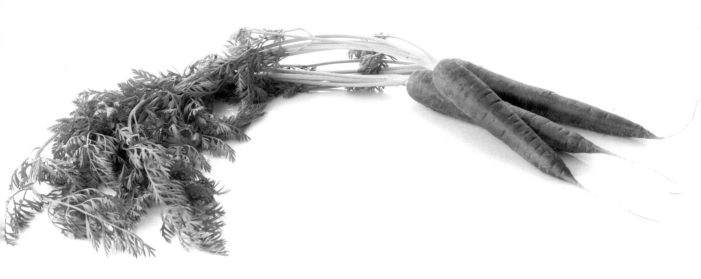

The Top Nine Vegetables of Choice for Your Healthy Smoothie

Here are the top nine vegetables of choice that I recommend starting with. The list is in no particular order:

Cucumber: A vegetable with a very high water content, the cucumber works best in savory recipes. Cucumbers are hydrating, refreshing, and a nice pick-me-up in smoothies. They are also rich in vitamins A, B1, B6, C, and D; folate; calcium; magnesium; and potassium. They add a mild taste to smoothies and help with weight loss and indigestion.

Broccoli: You may be hesitant to throw broccoli in at first. I was too. But broccoli is a true beauty food that nourishes your skin, as well as your internal joints and tissues with its high dose of minerals, including calcium, zinc, folate, and iron. I use the broccoli florets, not the thick stems, in smoothies, and you may just love the taste. Do try at least one recipe with broccoli.

Fennel: Fennel is a gorgeous vegetable with a big bulb and large stalks, and it smells heavenly. It is not cheap, so if you can get it now and again, it adds fragrance and a lift to your smoothies. A little goes a long way. It's crunchy, sweet, and refreshing, and both bulb and stem can be used in smoothies as a decent source of vitamin C.

Tomato: This red, lush, sweet, juicy vegetable (or fruit, depending on whom you ask) is great in all foods, including smoothies. Tomatoes are used in all the savory smoothies in this book. I like grapevine and heirloom tomatoes, but you can use whichever kind you like. Tomatoes are a big source of lycopene, and research suggests that they reduce the risk of cancer. Tomatoes are also high in vitamins A, C, and K.

Peppers: Peppers are a world of their own. I use them in some recipes here. You can always add a little hot pepper to any savory or even some sweet recipes, but always discard the seeds. All peppers are rich in vitamins A, C, and K, but red peppers are just bursting with them. Peppers also help with boosting your immune system, and you can get them in all flavors, from sweet to hot and super-hot.

Sweet potato: There are a couple of recipes with washed, peeled, cooked, and chilled sweet potato. Unlike regular potatoes, sweet potatoes have tons of nutrition and are very nice and filling. They are a great source of beta-carotene, much like carrots, and they taste, well, sweet. You get lots of vitamins and minerals and healthy starches from your sweet potatoes.

Cabbage: This crunchy vegetable is surprisingly mild as a base vegetable in smoothies with a great consistency. Ever had a cabbaggino at a Vitamix demo? You can only taste the coffee, none of the cabbage. Cabbage is also highly nutritious and a great source of Vitamin K. It's excellent for your digestion and surprisingly filling.

Carrots: Always buy your carrots with the carrot tops so you can use both for almost the same price. Carrots are excellent for your eyes and a great source of beta-carotene, which converts to vitamin A and many other nutrients, as well as being extremely delicious. Carrots go well in both sweet and savory recipes, and they lead to better vision, anti-aging effects, glowing skin, and they aid your body in flushing out the toxins.

Celery: This widely available and affordable vegetable is a darling and an excellent source of nutrition in your smoothies. Celery has a strong distinct taste, so always start with one stalk. It can help with puffiness and flushing out toxins from the body. Use the leaves of celery as well as the stalk. It's also a source of great minerals, calcium, magnesium, and potassium.

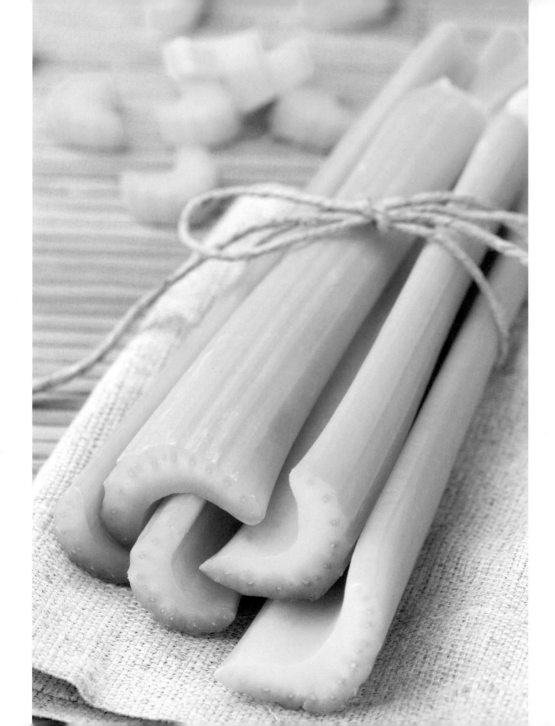

Amazing Medicinal Herbs to Add to Your Smoothie

What I call "medicinal herbs" are optional, of course. They give your smoothie a kick, a spice, and a wowza factor, but most of all, they give you a super dose of nutrition. I mainly use these three in my recipes in this book:

Garlic
Ginger
Cayenne pepper

What about using Green Powders instead of Fresh Greens in Your Smoothie?

If you don't have access to greens or vegetables, or if you are in a hurry and won't be able to grab that handful of fresh spinach, then you can use green powders

A green powder is the powdered form of select vegetables, generally the dark leafy vegetables. Because it's in powder form, most of the fiber has been extracted. Green powders are a form of superfood. Choose a powder that it is mostly organic and processed with protection from UV light and moisture, so that the good stuff—the chlorophyll and nutrients—are preserved as much as possible. Get quality powders that are raw and dehydrated. Store them in cool, dry places in your house to prevent exposure to light and heat, which can cause mold to grow. Avoid brands that have fillers like lecithin, fibers, whole grasses, pectin, rice bran, or flax. Go for pure organic green powder without extra stuff if possible.

All powders vary in taste and texture. They all smell differently too, but don't worry, you won't notice the smell in your smoothie. If you can grab small packets to sample it first, always do that before buying large containers of a product.

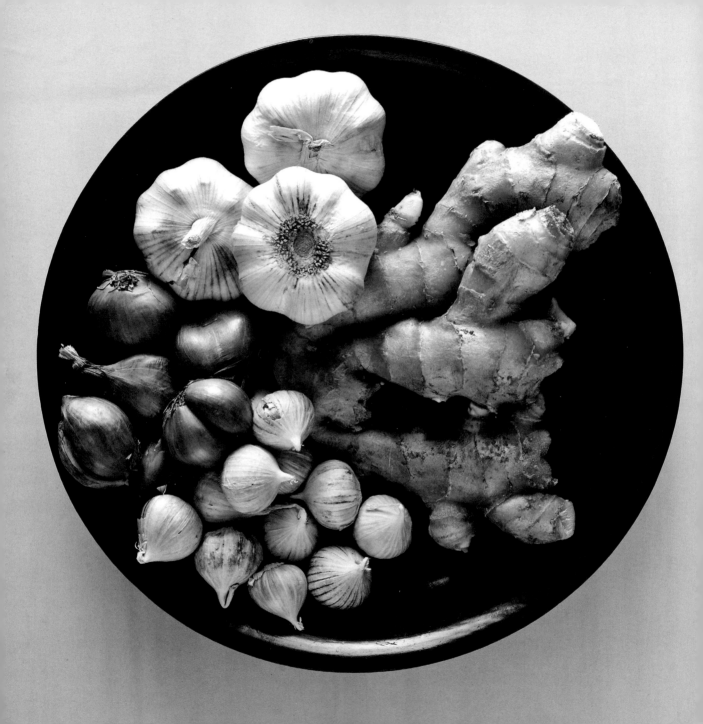

The Skinny on Fruits for Smoothies

When health is absent, wisdom cannot reveal itself, art cannot manifest, strength cannot fight, wealth becomes useless, and intelligence cannot be applied.
~Herophilus

Your base fruit is the primary fruit that gives the smoothie both its consistency and its majority taste. For your base, you want to choose at least a fruit that gives your smoothies that creamy, silky texture that holds it together. It binds the ingredients and makes it so much more delectable. These fruits are: banana, avocado, peach, mango, coconut, fig, and pear. Banana, avocado, and coconut give the creamiest texture. Avocado and coconut will also add natural good fats to your smoothie and make it more filling than bananas will. If you don't want to use fruit, you can use nut butters to give you this creamy binding texture.

Any other fruits that you use are flavor fruits. They are slightly lower in portion and they give an additional tang, sweetness, or tartness to your smoothie.

Fruit is the best companion to a green smoothie because it breaks down very quickly and digests well with leafy green vegetables. The effect of all this is best when you eat your green smoothies on an empty stomach. Breakfast is the ideal time for a smoothie.

All of the fruits in smoothies are fresh; never canned or in juiced form from bottles. Get your fruit in the produce section, or at farmer's markets to support your local community. I recommend buying your organic fruits as often as possible, and using them at their freshest. Fruit with a higher density, such as apples and pears, last longer than berries, so plan your shopping accordingly. Of course you can freeze most fruit to make it last longer, so grab it when you can get a good deal on the organic options, or buy more of what's in season. See the "Freezing Your Fruit" section in the next chapter for details.

The Top Twenty Fruits of Choice for Your Healthy Smoothie

Apple: An apple a day keeps the doctor away, right? This nutritious fruit, which is high in vitamins and minerals, is excellent for you. No need to peel your apples, but don't eat the seeds or the stem. Never freeze apples; always use fresh ones in smoothies. You can choose any type of apple that you like. Just note that green apples are sour, so if you want the apple to act as a sweetener in your smoothie, use yellow or Fuji apples.

Avocado: One day, I want to own avocado trees. This gorgeous, creamy little delight is a source of excellent fat and vitamins for your body, is extremely filling, and goes very well as a base fruit in your smoothies. It is very low in sugar and adds a great texture to smoothies. The skin and pit are inedible. Oh, and as far as protein goes, avocados have all eighteen essential amino acids to be a complete protein food. Good news if you're cutting out meat!

Banana: The universal magical fruit that works fine in just about any smoothie, combines well with almost all flavors, and is oh-so-affordable. I remember when I lived in Iran, bananas were rare and such a treat. Bananas are full of nutrition and benefits for your body and mind—they help you overcome depression, thanks to their generous levels of serotonin! Bananas can also help with indigestion, alertness, and controlling your sugar cravings. Have bananas handy at all times!

Berries (Blueberries, Strawberries, Raspberries, Blackberries, Cranberries, Grapes): Tiny, tasty, and tantalizingly colorful, berries are also powerful allies for your health, protecting everything from your head to your heart. These antioxidant-rich little fruits are also low in sugar and mix wonderfully with the leafy greens. The recipes in this book use a mix of these berries, fresh or frozen. You can also explore additional berries. Berries play a big role in the eventual color of your smoothie!

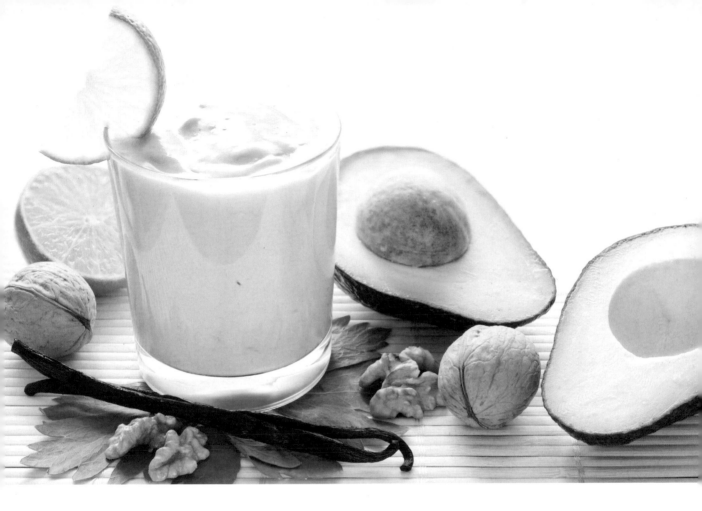

Coconut: This delicious, multi-purpose wonder fruit can be a heavenly addition to your smoothies in the form of coconut milk, meat, and even oil, although oil is very high in fat and not included in any of my recipes. Did you know that during World War II in some cases medics would siphon pure coconut water from young coconuts to be used as emergency plasma transfusions for soldiers who were injured? Coconut water is that pure . . . wowza! Learn how to knock a coconut open and use it in your smoothies.

Fig: The queen of all fruits to me, the fig is an ancient fruit from Asia that is exquisite in taste and texture, and it is a tremendous addition to any smoothie. Did you know that the Romans would give each other presents of figs on the first day of their new year? And fun fig religion factoids: Biblical tradition holds that Adam and Eve covered their nakedness with the leaves of the fig tree as they were expelled from heaven. And in Buddhism, the fig tree is a symbol of enlightenment. It is believed that the Buddha achieved enlightenment while sitting under a Bodhi tree (which is a type of fig tree). Buy fresh figs and freeze them. They are not cheap, but for this one, I'd say you're worth the luxury!

Kiwi: I admit, I am not a big fan of kiwi, but this little fruit has more vitamin C than its other citrus cousins and is a popular addition to smoothies. Kiwi needs to be peeled, but can be used fresh or frozen. It helps boost your immunity, improve your digestive system, and regulate blood sugar. Use it as you desire.

Lemon: The fruit with a hundred purposes, I rub the juice of a fresh lemon on my skin as a wonderful face "mask," put it in my water and salads, or juice it through a juicer and use fresh juice of lemon in smoothies. The ancient Romans believed that lemons helped your body fight off poison. Lemons are excellent for you, and a few drops of juice helps a smoothie last longer in the fridge. Always have a lemon handy!

Lime: Lemon's sibling, lime has very similar properties to lemon, but I have used it in only a select number of smoothies. It does wonders in the savory ones.

Mango: An excellent base fruit for your smoothies, mangos are great both fresh and frozen. They give your smoothies a nice creamy texture and tons of nutrition, vitamins, and minerals, plus acts as a skin cleanser, and the fiber-rich nature of this yellow fruit fills you up. Peel and de-core them and get them ready for use!

Orange: Did you know orange and spinach go together like bread and butter? Me neither! But they do! Orange is a universally loved fruit, and you already know it's a

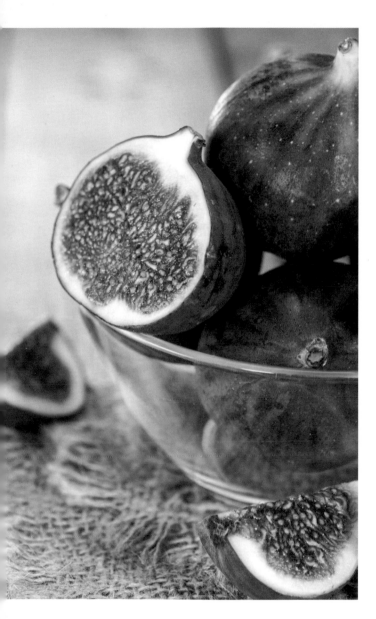

powerhouse of nutrition, antioxidants, and good for you. Using it in smoothies is fun; the citrus taste cuts down the bitterness of greens. Use your oranges fresh and peel them right before using, but no earlier. Never eat the peels!

Pear: Pears are a great source of fiber, have a wealth of vitamins and minerals, are relatively low in sugar, and can be a great base fruit in smoothies. Never freeze your pears. Always use fresh ones, and use the whole pear, except the seeds and stem. They are relatively inexpensive, so you can treat yourself to this one often.

Pineapple: If only this sweet juicy delicious darling was not so hard to peel! Pineapples are delicious, and can turn a super-green and bitter smoothie into a party you don't want to miss. They are great if you are warding off colds, and they're good for your gums and bones. They also act as a natural inflammatory for the body, so they help with the healing of bruises and injuries, too. Be sure to peel your pineapple completely and discard the hard middle section.

Peach: Fresh or frozen, this widely adored fruit originates from China and is perfect for your smoothies—and it comes with tons of nutrition to boot. Peaches are great for relieving stress, fighting cancer, weight loss, and as with most other fruits, they're full of vitamins and antioxidants.

Pomegranate: This beautiful, rich red fruit is the symbol of fertility in China and a staple in Persian cuisine. The health benefits of the pomegranate are numerous. The queen of antioxidants, pomegranate is also excellent for digestion, bladder problems, skin, circulation, weight loss, and inflammation. Pomegranates are not cheap, so treat yourself when you can. The seeds are juicy little jewels—bright red, tart, and crunchy. The problem is, they're encased in a hard, tight skin, which, although lovely to look at, is difficult to break into. The magic trick is to first cut the fruit in half and next cut it in quarters. Then put the quarters in a bowl of cold water and gently nudge the seeds away from the skin with your fingers right under the water. No muss! No fuss! Now you don't have an excuse not to buy pomegranates.

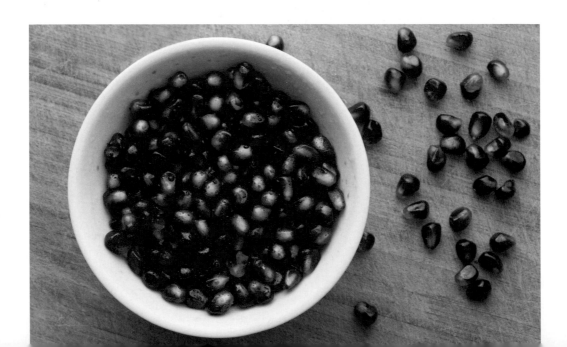

Leslie Broberg

Favorite Recipe: Spiced Tropical Kale Smoothie

½ fresh or frozen banana
1 cup ice (less if using frozen banana)
3 leaves of any kale, or more to taste, without the stems
1 cup unsweetened coconut or vanilla almond milk
½ to 1 serving protein powder
1 tbsp unsweetened shredded coconut
1 dash of nutmeg
1 dash of cinnamon

Place the ice and banana at the bottom of the blender, then add the other ingredients. Blend until smooth at medium speed. Serve.

This recipe was a perfect solution to two problems: What to have for breakfast if you find breakfast food boring, and how to get some kale in there, the last frontier for me in terms of green foods. I find kale a bit strong, but this recipe has lots of other flavors. Note the use of nutmeg in the recipe, which is a classic Italian addition to many of the green foods they prepare at home. It just helps to offset the bitterness of greens.

Leslie Broberg is a self-professed foodie who became a paid personal chef at the age of 15, and went on to become a journalist and editor in the science sector. She loves a good restaurant, but these days she's cooking more meals at home. It really makes a difference when you cook your own healthy food, she says, and there are many healthy and tasty recipes out there that do not take long to prepare. As a blogger, she shares some of her experiences at iwantavitamix.com.

On Superfoods, Seeds, and Powders

Attention to health is life's greatest hindrance.
~Plato

What is a superfood anyway? Some would say "superfood" is a marketing term used to describe foods with supposed health benefits. Superfood is a nutritionally dense food with particular health benefits. This is a very popular term in the health industry right now. Frankly, all fruits and vegetables, especially leafy greens, are a type of superfood. They are superior to just about any other choice you could make in your daily nutritional choices, even if they don't come packaged with a stamp of approval from some company.

Superfood can mean a lot of things. If you research the term, you will find dozens of different lists on websites, and you'll find anything on the lists from apples to legumes to oats to berries to fish to yogurt! Each list highlights one angle of the nutritional benefits of that particular food. All of those foods can be great for you, yes, and you can add them to your diet in moderation and enjoy the benefits. But the superfoods we talk about with regard to smoothies are obviously not in the legume or dairy category!

I define superfoods as the rarer fruits, vegetables, or greens in a densely concentrated form that give you a great nutritional edge over other foods. They are whole foods that have been cultivated without altering the form, without adding pesticides or chemicals, and with excellent nutritional profiles. They are natural foods, even though they may come "packaged." You won't find them in your produce section, as you would the regular fruits and vegetables, but most health food stores carry them.

Green smoothies are the easiest and most hidden vehicle to sneak those superfoods into your body. You can add goji berries and acai berry powder for extra protein and a

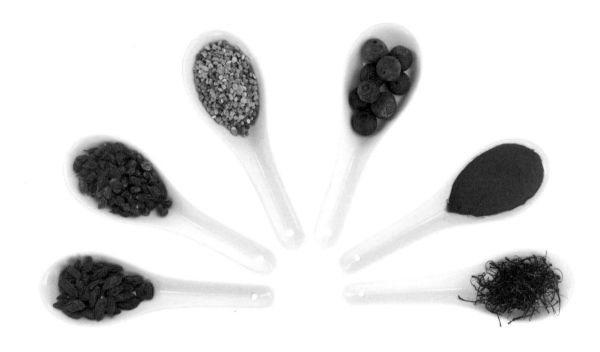

high dose of antioxidants, flaxseed powder and chia seeds for a boost of your plant-based omega-3 fatty acids, and raw cacao and maca root powders for an energy boost—not to mention delicious, distinct taste.

First things first: You do not *need* superfoods. You can add them into your smoothies, and that's what this section talks about, but you can just as easily skip them and rely on the powers of a handful of fruits and vegetables to bring you a powerhouse of nutrition, minerals, vitamins, and other goodies. My goal is to make healthy smoothies accessible as well as affordable for you, and relying on exotic, hard-to-find, and often expensive ingredients is not the way to go about it.

A majority of the recipes in this book are written in such a way that if you never want to use a single superfood, you are fine. You can get great taste and excellent nutrition without fancy, expensive, and exotic powders, and I make plenty of delicious smoothies that way on a regular basis.

Now having said that, superfoods add a lot of fun, spice, variety, and flavor to your smoothie, plus the aforementioned edge on the nutrition scale. So if you have the means, I say experiment. I have tested many different superfoods and have a recommendation of the "Top Products of Choice" in the next section to help you decide which to use.

Make sure you keep all your superfoods in tightly lidded containers and store them in a cool place—no need to put in your fridge, the pantry will do, unless you have ground up your own flaxseed powder, which is best refrigerated.

Here are the specific superfoods that I enjoy using and have included in the recipes in this book. You can find most of these relatively easily at most health food stores, or order them online:

1. **Goji berries:** These beautiful, dark red berries, which are usually found in dried, packaged form, are a true superfood, plus they're tasty. They have healthy fats, soluble fiber, a huge dose of antioxidants, and some trace minerals, such as zinc, iron, and phosphorus. They are said to have more vitamin C than their orange cousins, and more beta-carotene than carrots. The taste is what keeps you coming back to them. My favorite go-to brand for goji berries is Navitas Naturals.

2. **Flaxseed powder:** Use flaxseeds in a ground form only. A spoonful of flaxseed powder (also known as flaxseed meal) gives you a boost of essential fatty acids, especially omega-3s. They have a high dose of fiber and a very mild nutty flavor, plus the usual goodness of vitamin and minerals. You get vitamin B6, calcium, magnesium, folate, and

iron from these seeds. I love the Navitas Naturals brand, which is gluten-free, vegan, and organic. You can add flaxseed powder to just about any non-savory smoothie.

3. **Acai powder:** This deep, dark purple-colored powder adds a wonderful berry flavor to your breakfast smoothies, and it is rich with antioxidants, anti-inflammatory, and anti-cancer properties, plus a great source for your fatty acids, fiber, protein, and so much more. It originates from the Amazon rainforest and is one of the foods that the indigenous cultures depend on as a source of their sustenance and good health. Again, my favorite brand is Navitas Naturals.

4. **Hemp seeds and hemp powder:** You can get these in powder or seed form. I do love the seeds, and my favorite brand is Hemp Hearts by Manitoba Harvest, which has a lovely nutty flavor and very slight crunch. The seeds do not need to be ground for your smoothie, so you can use either powder or seed form. They are a great source of plant-based protein, omega-6, and omega-3 essential fatty acids. Much like flaxseed powder, you can add hemp seeds or powder to just about non-savory smoothie. Hemp is one of the best foods to build strong and lean muscle.

5. **Chia seeds:** You can enjoy these in their black seed form or in the sprouted, finely milled powder form, and my go-to brand is the latter by Navitas Naturals. These seeds come from Central America, where they are used in food and medicine, and they are abundant in omega fats, protein, antioxidants, vitamin B12, folate, and dietary fiber. They are an excellent source of workout food, give you lots of energy, and provide strengthening and toning nutrients. Again, these lovely seeds add taste and texture and go in most non-savory and breakfast smoothies.

6. **Sesame seeds:** An ancient seed from the old east, sesame seeds are a beautifully nutritious seed and a great source of trace minerals such as iron, zinc, magnesium, manganese, and copper, not to mention a great source of vitamins and fiber. I love raw sesame

seeds, but you can get them toasted, too. The taste of sesame seeds makes them one of my favorites. You can add sesame seeds to just about any smoothie, savory or not.

7. **Sunflower seeds:** These delicious seeds, which can serve as a perfect snack on their own, promote glowing skin. They also contain the trace minerals copper, phosphorus, and selenium, as well as being a great source of vitamin E, vitamins B1 and B5, fiber, and folate—but that's not all. They are a powerhouse of nutrition, make any smoothie more delicious, and can even calm anxiety and promote relaxation for the brain. Don't forget to add these into your smoothies once in a while!

8. **Cacao powder:** A taste that once you try, you'll never want to live without—at least, I haven't, not since my hubby whipped up a gluten-free, vegan, raw "brownie" recipe during my vegan phase. Cacao powder makes delicious dessert smoothies, among other types. As soon as you start using cacao powder, you'll associate the taste of chocolate with this refined beauty, and you might even lose your taste for regular candy or "chocolate" bars, which are not good for you. Cacao powder is also a great source of antioxidants and has an abundance of magnesium and iron. Try to get it in raw form. My go-to brand here is most definitely Navitas Naturals.

9. **Matcha Green tea:** Matcha is a finely ground, powdered, high-quality green tea. This tea is not the same as regular tea powder or green tea powder. This bitter, strong, and gorgeous tea from ancient Japan has even more benefits for you than regular green tea. It is full of antioxidants, helps with digestion, provides an energy boost, and detoxes, but that's not all. Matcha contains a potent class of antioxidant known as catechin that is not easily found in any other foods, and one that has great cancer-fighting abilities. Use it sparingly, starting with ¼ of a teaspoon.

10. **Spirulina:** Coming from the blue-green algae family, it is full of phytonutrients, a great source of protein, and best in powdered form. This is one of the superfoods that will take some time to get used to—it has a very particular taste, so start with small

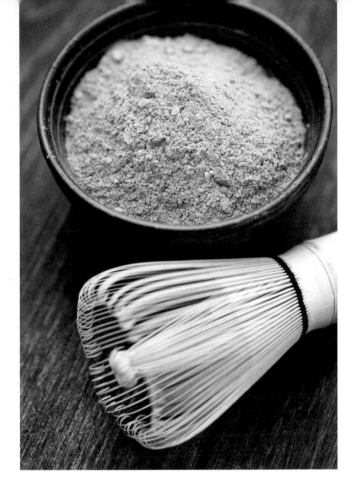

amounts and add more over time. It has a rich green taste to it and a little goes a long way, but it's an excellent food. Spirulina is known to help stamina and even curb hunger. You can add as little as ½ teaspoon to your smoothie of choice and still get plenty of benefits. Oh, and no matter what your smoothie, spirulina turns it into this gorgeous, deep blue-green ocean color. It's like magic.

Should You Add Protein Powders to Your Smoothie?

You certainly can. All the protein powders tested here are vegan and among the highest brands. I would encourage you to check the ingredients in your protein powder, and make sure it is a high-quality brand with favorable customer reviews. Raw vegan protein powders derived from brown rice, sprouts, or other non-soy plants are good choices.

Remember, you do not need to use protein powders to get a complete meal from your healthy smoothie. You get plenty of protein from nut butters, nut milks, chia seeds, flaxseeds, or hemp seeds, as well as leafy greens and other types of vegetables. These are more natural and better sources of protein for your body. However, if you are athletic or want to build muscle, or just want additional protein and calories in your smoothie to make it into a fuller meal, go for it.

Recommended Brands for Select Products

To give you a head-start with some of the superfoods listed above, as well as the protein powders and other additions to your smoothies, I have compiled some of my favorite brands. By no means is this a comprehensive list, as there are a lot of companies putting out tasty (and healthy!) accompaniments for your smoothies.

Remember that these are based on personal taste, so don't be afraid to experiment.

Recommended Brands of Products

Product	Recommendation	Why?
Goji berries	Navitas Naturals Goji Berries	Excellent goji berries, great taste in smoothie, great price.
Flaxseed powder	Navitas Naturals Organic Flaxseed Sprouted Powder	Easiest to digest, highest quality, and (almost) odor-free.
Acai powder	Navitas Naturals Organic Acai Powder	Super-fine powder, highest quality, nice packaging.
Hemp seeds / powder	Manitoba Harvest Hemp Seed Nut	Highest quality hemp seeds, nutty flavor, nice packaging, great taste and price.
Chia seed powder	Navitas Naturals Chia Seed Sprouted Powder	Prefer powder to seeds for chia; this finely ground powder is delicious.
Cacao powder	Navitas Naturals Organic Raw Cacao Powder	BEST cacao powder, highest quality, organic, raw, simply delectable.
Matcha Green tea	Organic Ceremonial Matcha by DoMatcha	Excellent fine powdered Matcha, great price, great packaging to keep fresh.
Spirulina	Nutrex Hawaii Hawaiian Spirulina Powder	Excellent source of spirulina, trusted brand, high quality, great price.
Oats	Bob's Red Mill Gluten-Free Rolled Oats	Highest quality, most delicious oats, soaks brilliantly, trusted brand.
Powdered Smoothie Mix	Green Power Organic Superfood Blend by GreenLifeFood	Great blend of greens, veggies, and superfoods including wheatgrass; raw, organic, works well with fruit smoothies.

Product	Recommendation	Why?
Powdered Smoothie Mix	Amazing Meal Chocolate Infusion by Amazing Grass	Nutrition values high, sugar low, taste is great, blends really well in smoothie, no gritty or grainy texture, yummy aftertaste.
Powdered Smoothie Mix	Amazing Meal Vanilla Chai Infusion by Amazing Grass	Delicious taste, low sugar, mixes well, cuts bitterness of greens, great source of protein.
Powdered Smoothie Mix	BerryRadical Antioxidant Superfood by Miessence	Super high-quality source of antioxidants, trusted brand, natural ingredients.
Powdered Smoothie Mix	InLiven Probiotic Superfood by Miessence	Super high-quality source of probiotics, trusted brand, natural ingredients.
Vegan Protein Powder	Living Harvest Organic Hemp Protein Powder, Original Flavor	Trusted brand, great source of protein, does not alter taste of smoothie, easy to digest.
Vegan Protein Powder	Living Harvest Organic Hemp Protein Powder, Vanilla Chai	Very tasty and great source of protein, trusted brand, excellent flavor, low in sugar.
Vegan Protein Powder	Raw Power Protein Mix, Original Flavor	Excellent protein powder, mixes well in all smoothies, tasteless, super-easy to digest.
Vegan Protein Powder	Raw Power Raw Warrior Brown Rice Protein Powder	Delicious protein powder for all smoothies, top-notch brand, love this product.
Protein Powder	Standard Process SP Complete Dairy Free	Trusted brand, highly tested, great source of protein, tasteless, easy to digest.
Vegan Protein Powder	Sunwarrior Warrior Blend Raw Protein	Delicious and great source of protein, great price, serving size perfect, easy to digest.

Vickie Velasquez

Favorite Recipe: Vickie's Summer Spirulina Smoothie

$\frac{2}{3}$ cup soy milk
$\frac{1}{3}$ cup coconut water
1 banana, cut into pieces
1 cup torn kale
1 cup spinach leaves
1 cup strawberries, stems and leaves removed
1 tbsp ground flaxseed
1 tbsp spirulina powder
4 ice cubes

Vickie Velasquez became a vegetarian in January of 2013. She began a podcast and website, Vegetarian Zen (vegetarianzen.com), with her partner, Larissa Galenes, in order to help others understand the many benefits of a diet rich in plant-based foods. Most of her followers are not vegetarians, but rather call themselves "veg-curious" and want to make healthier eating choices overall. She is out to help them! She was inspired to create this smoothie after a hard workout of cardio and resistance training. She knew she wanted to get protein into her body to help repair her muscles, so she reached for the spirulina, spinach, and kale but because it was also a hot South Texas summer day when she created this drink, she wanted something with a refreshing tropical taste—hence the bananas, strawberries, and coconut water.

Choosing Your Liquid Base

The greatest of follies is to sacrifice health for any other kind of happiness.
~Arthur Schweitzer

Your smoothie will need a liquid base to help the blending process, as well as to add extra flavor as an optional bonus. You must add some liquid, not just to get the right smoothie texture, but to also avoid damaging the blender motor.

The easiest base to use is filtered water. You can use this base in every smoothie recipe if you wish. I use room-temperature tap water that has been filtered. You can use any filtered water. I avoid bottled water for many reasons, but the main one is that I find the taste of filtered water to be the most pleasing. It's just a personal preference, plus using bottled water gets expensive and inconvenient. I also use room-temperature water because the frozen fruit adds the coldness factor to the smoothie already.

If you want to add more density and some flavor to your smoothie, you have many fun and delicious options.

Nut milks are a great creamy, filling liquid base for your smoothie. You can use half nut milk and half water to mix it up and to dilute the creamier smoothies. On some occasions, I also use freshly squeezed juice. You can mix juice with your smoothie, but I highly recommend you press it fresh in your own kitchen and avoid buying bottled juices.

You can either buy nut milk or make nut milks at home with a high-powered blender, such as the Vitamix or the Blendtec, and a food processor. Homemade nut milks are delicious, but I personally buy my nut milks at Whole Foods to save time and hassle. I like the Silk, Blue Diamond, and Califia brands best. When choosing nut milks, I like those that are fortified with calcium and vitamin D, which helps the absorption of calcium. Just check the ingredients to see if your brand of choice offers this. I also always choose unsweetened. The additional flavoring adds extra sugar and possibly food coloring, which is not good for you.

I avoid soy milk because it's lower in nutrition and personally I don't find it to be tasty. However, the real reason I don't use it is because there are controversial studies about soy, and a large number of them claim that soy is not good for your health and can even be detrimental. So why chance it? It doesn't taste that good—to me, anyway—and you have so many healthier and more delicious options. My two cents'? Skip soy milk!

You can also modify. If a recipe calls for almond milk, you can use half that amount of almond milk and the other half just filtered water if you want a lighter smoothie—or vice versa, if the recipe calls for filtered water, you can use coconut water to enrich the taste without adding too much of a change in flavor.

Here are the smoothie bases used in this book:

Filtered water: I use a Brita filter to filter tap water and keep it at room temperature. Filtered water is the base of all my savory recipes, plus a few non-savory ones, and it makes a perfect base for your own future smoothie concoctions, too!

Almond Milk: Unsweetened almond milk is my favorite non-water base. You can buy it at regular grocery stores these days. Make sure you get unsweetened and unflavored. The flavored ones usually have extra sugar.

Coconut Milk: Unsweetened coconut milk is another favorite base, especially when mixed with pineapple! Coconut milk is the liquid that comes from the grated meat of a coconut. The color and rich taste of the milk can be attributed to the high oil content. Most of the fat is saturated fat. Coconut milk goes a long way. Again, get the unsweetened version.

Coconut Water: Coconut water is the clear liquid inside young coconuts. It is not as dense and does not contain the high fat content of coconut milk, but it is still more substantial than filtered water, so if you want to replace plain water with something more but don't want to use nut milk, this is a great median between the two.

Almond-Coconut Milk: A lot of brands that have almond or coconut milk also have a combination, and I use this one a lot, too. It has a rich nutty flavor and you get the nutrients from both almonds and coconuts. Opt for the unsweetened version and feel free to replace this delicious combo with any other nut milks in the recipes.

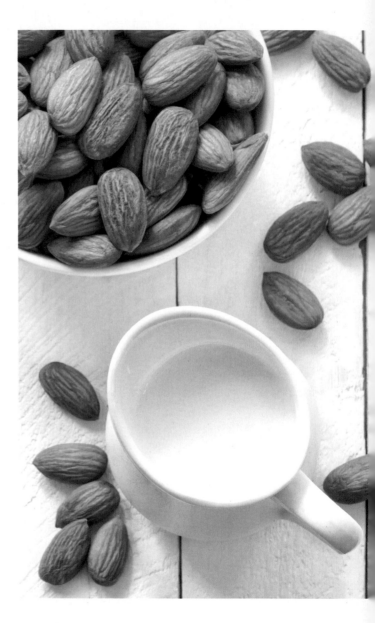

Matcha Green Tea: Matcha tea is not just any tea. It is a top antioxidant machine of a superfood. You could add just a half or full teaspoon of tea powder with a water base, but the best way would be to properly make the Matcha tea first, then let it chill in the refrigerator. To make tea, measure out one teaspoon of matcha into a matcha bowl. Let 1½ cups of boiling water sit for five minutes to cool down before you pour the water into the bowl. Then whisk the mixture rapidly until the tea is dissolved and the liquid is topped with a light-colored foam. It's normal for some of the powder to remain at the bottom of the bowl. Chill in the fridge, and you've got your base for your next smoothie.

Hemp milk: This is not one of my regular choices for a base because I like getting my hemp in the form of seeds, but if this is your favorite, use it. Living Harvest has a very good brand called Tempt Hemp, which I have enjoyed.

Cashew Milk: Not as common in grocery stores, and one that you would probably need to make at home, but if you really like the flavor of cashews, this is a nut milk you can make using your food processor or a high-powered blender. Cashews are a lot less expensive than almonds, and if you make your own, you may just come out ahead on the spending scale.

Rice Milk: This is the mildest-tasting and lowest nutrient choice among the non-dairy milks. I have used it enough to know that I don't care for the taste or the nutritional value, and I do not recommend it, unless you are in an absolute pinch.

You can also use fresh squeezed or store-bought juice that is cold-pressed, never-heated, and with nothing added to it. I did not add this as a base in my recipes, because it's a double effort to use both the juicer and the blender to make your smoothie, but if you made some fresh carrot or orange juice earlier in the day or even yesterday, feel free to get creative!

On Mixing and Matching Flavors

Put your brain into gear before you put your mouth into motion.
~Unknown

Mixing and matching the flavors in your smoothie is a lot of fun, but it takes a little while to get the hang of it. With all recipes, you will have a base fruit as well as a flavor fruit. The base fruit is what you will primarily taste in your smoothie, and the flavor fruit(s) are what you add to give the smoothie the extra flavors and boost the overall nutritional profile of your drink.

Flavor fruits are totally optional, but I highly recommend you add them in. They especially enhance the overall taste of a green smoothie and cut down the bitterness and strong flavor of greens.

Here are some ideas on what base fruits and flavor fruits combine extremely well together. Remember, this is not the only way to combine fruits by any stretch of imagination. These are simply combinations that I enjoy and have used in some of the recipes here, and it's just to get you started. You can use these or create your own by mixing and matching flavors and explore to your heart's content.

Wildly delicious base and flavor fruit combos:

Banana with any berry
Banana with pear
Avocado with pineapple
Avocado with pear
Avocado with pomegranate
Mango with pineapple
Mango with pomegranate
Peach with strawberry
Pear with apple

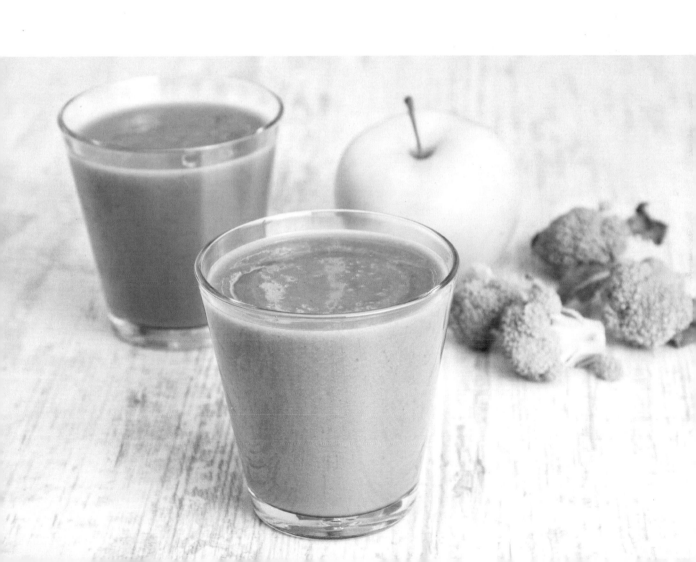

You can add additional flavors with the superfoods, herbs, and spices. You could also add protein powders if desired. Just use neutral powders to keep the fruit tastes intact. If you want to add even more flavors in each sip (or spoonful), add fun ingredients, such as cacao, goji berries, and spices like vanilla and cinnamon.

Sometimes you may want a simpler recipe. Sometimes you want fun and adventure in your glass. Sometimes I just want three flavors in my smoothie and some greens. Other times, I want something fun and complex. As you learn to listen to your moods and your cravings, you'll find the best way to respond to them with smoothie magic!

Remember that you can add extra flavor by including a dash of cinnamon, nutmeg, pumpkin spice, vanilla extract, or a vanilla bean to any recipe.

What Not to Add to Your Smoothies

It is easier to change a man's religion than to change his diet.
~Margaret Mead

Never add table sugar, artificial sweeteners, corn or other syrups, or any refined foods to your healthy smoothies.

You do not want to waste all your efforts of creating a perfectly healthy drink! Use natural ways to sweeten your smoothie, such as increasing the dosage of your fresh fruit base. If you want to go even sweeter, then add a very small amount of raw honey or some dried fruit, such as dates or figs—but aim to sweeten your drink with fresh fruit first. Use raw honey as a last resort to sweeten your smoothie if fruits don't do the job.

Powdered sweeteners, such as stevia or Splenda, and syrups like agave are not good for you, and the whole point of smoothies is to help you cut your cravings for those processed sugars, not increase your desire for them! This is a process of changing and adapting your taste buds to higher quality levels of sweetness.

Your smoothies will be sweet enough with just fruit, and if you want to sweeten them even more to your taste, especially as you first get started, you can increase your fruit dosage. Use fruit to adjust your taste buds to the natural flavors of sugar and gradually wean yourself off the sugar addiction. That's one of the powerful benefits of smoothies—you can train your taste buds to appreciate the natural flavors of fruits and vegetables, and not lust after artificial sugars. Just be patient with yourself and you'll notice this benefit over time. Stick to nature's own sweeteners to get just the right taste for your smoothie.

Adrienne Jurado

Favorite Recipe: Not-So Piña Colada

8 oz kefir (plain, unsweetened, preferably homemade)
1 tbsp virgin coconut oil
1 banana (medium ripe)
1 ½–2 cups spinach
1 cup of strawberries
1 cup of ice (½ cup if using frozen strawberries)
I tsp Honey (Optional)

Adrienne's turning point began in an unexpected way about three years ago. She attended a friend's party for a beauty-product line. She was shocked to discover how many chemicals go into everyday skincare products. She swore off them for good and started making her own beauty care products. Then she realized that if what she's putting on her body is so important to her health, what she's putting in her body deserves even more attention. This turned into a major overhaul of her diet, which is now mostly grass-fed and free-range sources of meat, vegetables, fruits, nuts, and healthy fats. She tried to jump on the green smoothie bandwagon, but repeatedly failed until they bought a high-quality blender. Now they enjoy a delicious green smoothie nearly every day.

The "Not-So Piña Colada" is super simple, as well as a beach-time favorite. She can't believe how much this smoothie reminds her of a real piña colada, even without the pineapple, a guilt-free delight.

Adrienne Jurado is a yoga teacher, experiential teambuilding facilitator, and blogger with a background in physics, psychology, military service, and outdoor leadership. She makes yoga more accessible to beginners by keeping it simple and enjoyable at her online yoga and wellness community, YOGADRIENNE.com.

In the Kitchen: Getting Ready to Blend

The beauty of smoothies is how very easy they are to make. Just about every kitchen boasts a blender of some sort, a knife, a fridge, and a power plug. You now have the basic tools of the smoothie-making trade. The reason I go into detail here is to make the process even faster, better, and more efficient, because there are several factors that affect this.

First, the type of blender you choose will directly affect the resulting smoothie, and it will also determine how fun and easy versus inconvenient it is to make that smoothie. You do not need a $500 power blender, but you do need a good one.

Secondly, how you go about the shopping, washing, storage, and preparation of your smoothie makes a huge impact on whether you keep it up or let it go. You may have a lot of time to think about that and to follow the natural rhythms of your schedule. If so, you won't need this section, but most of us are very busy, and every level of preparation can save more time and make it more enjoyable to keep making these smoothies.

Your goal here is to remove any and all barriers, even one as small as replacing a dull knife with a sharp one or buying some higher quality zip-top bags to store your frozen fruit. You need to take most of these preparation steps once and then you are set, but neglecting them could take up time and lead to frustration down the road.

Don't let that happen. Smoothies can be so much fun! Let's get savvy with the business of making irresistibly delicious and healthy smoothies today!

Smoothie Tools of the Trade

No disease that can be treated by diet should be treated with any other means.
~Maimonides

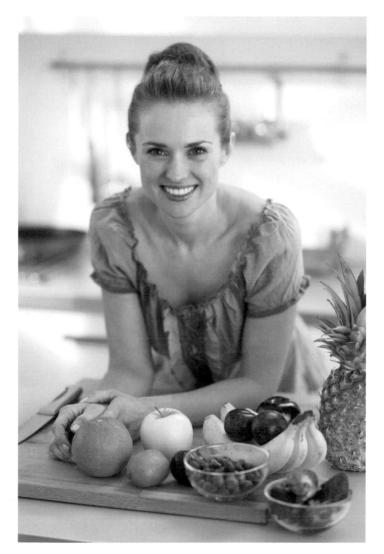

The barrier to entry into the world of smoothies is very low. You need so little to equip yourself to make these delicious smoothies that you would be silly not to, and you do not need an expertise in nutrition or medicine to be very good at it. Making healthy smoothies is an art that anybody can learn. In fact, at a minimum, you need a blender, and that is all. You can make do with everything else if you just have a blender. In the next section, I'll help you select the best blender for your needs and budget. Here's everything else that can make your smoothie process fun, easy, quick, and streamlined:

1. **A sharp knife or a knife set:** You are going to be cutting a lot of fruits and vegetables. Dull knives slow down everything, have a higher risk of injury, and are a waste of your precious time. Invest in at least one good, sharp knife.

2. **A cutting board:** I like the bamboo cutting boards, but you can get whatever you like. Just don't do the cutting on your counters. Protect them by always using a cutting board.

3. **Refrigerator and freezer:** I know this is mostly a given, but remember that you need to store your fruits and greens somewhere cold. A freezer is necessary to freeze all your fruit. If not frozen, bananas can be left out at room temperature.

4. **Access to a grocery store and/or farmer's market:** I was surprised how little I knew about the variety of grocery stores within a five-mile radius of my house. If you always go to the same place, look up other options. Indian or Asian grocery stores have some greens, vegetables, and fruits at very reasonable prices. Farmer's markets give you access to local produce, which is always fresher.

5. **Optional: Access to a health food store or ability to shop Amazon or other online stores:** If you want to get superfoods or protein powders, this would come in handy. It is a nice-to-have, and you do not need to regularly frequent such a place. I buy most of my superfoods and protein powders online or at Whole Foods, and I do watch my budget. Superfoods and protein powders are optional. Your green smoothie with greens and fruits is your superfood!

Selecting the Best Blender for You

Each patient carries his own doctor inside him.
~Norman Cousins

I have broken more than my fair share of blenders. There was that first cheap $17 blender I got at Wal-Mart. The motor died shortly after, smoke and all. Then I upgraded to an Oster blender. The motor also died, but this time with no smoke. Then the nice $200+ Breville blender that did not have the horsepower necessary to blend frozen fruit. It did not make the smoothies as creamy in texture as I would have liked. I gave it away because it wouldn't break on me.

Now, I live and die by my Vitamix. I love the Vitamix, and I am never looking back, except maybe to try the Blendtec, which is the other high-powered blender on the market competing neck-in-neck with the Vitamix. With a $500 to $600 price range, these power blenders are pricey, but they can become your staple kitchen appliance for years, and get used several times per day, not to mention for multiple purposes—I love making soups in addition to smoothies using the Vitamix, and I truly believe I am saving money by having a high-quality blender with multiple purposes.

Having said that, I've made some impressive smoothies in the Magic Bullet, and it works just fine. Both the Nutri Bullet and Magic Bullet brands are sturdy, boast a strong engine for their size and price range, and yield creamy, delicious smoothies. You also have the advantage of not having to pour out your smoothie into another glass. You just turn over the hard plastic cup container in which you blended, put the cap on, and you're all set. Their plastic cups fit nicely in most cupholders. I love those little machines. They travel very well in case you want to take your smoothie along with you on the road.

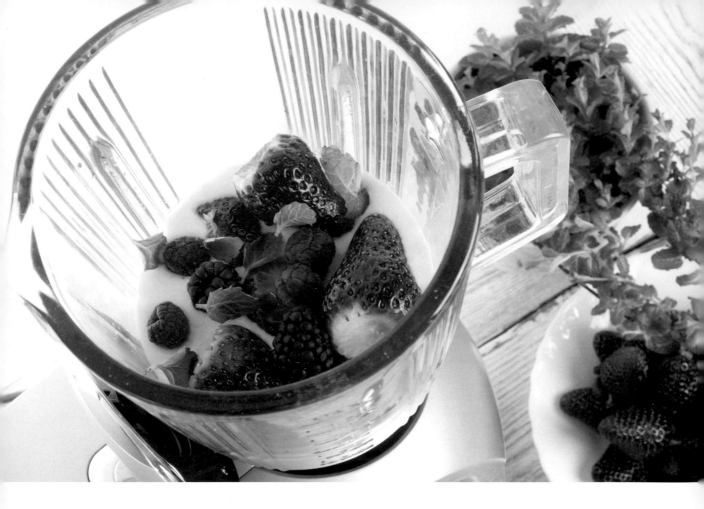

When you are choosing your blender, what matters is how well the machine blends and what quality of smoothie it produces. The higher the motor power, the better it can blend and handle the frozen items, and it will last longer despite frequent use. If you can produce high-quality smoothies that are fully blended, creamy, and smooth, as if you ordered it at a high-end restaurant, you are likely to continue making them. The whole point is to establish this as a habit, so keep that in mind as you shop for your blender.

A few things to pay attention to when choosing your blender:

1. **Amazon and other website reviews:** Always do your research. Amazon is a great place not just to shop, but also to do extensive research. My rule of thumb is to buy products that have an overwhelming number of four- and five-star reviews, with at least a few one- or two-star reviews. Note that I said with at least a few poor reviews—it always makes me think twice when a product has 100 five-star reviews; it's possible some of those may have been endorsed. Skim the reviews for obvious patterns and learn the pros and cons of the product as you do. If someone got their shipment late or a random chipped product was shipped out, it's likely an anomaly and not a pattern. But if ten people write about a motor breaking after the machine's third use, I'd move on to the next brand fast.

2. **Warranty quality and extent:** When you find a good brand that has a solid number of positive reviews and fits your price range, check on the warranty. The length and quality of the warranty is a big purchasing decision for me. I would gladly pay a little more for two or three more years of full coverage. The idea is to buy a machine that lasts you at least three to five years without breaking down, creates smooth and creamy blends, and fits your budget. Also note that if you pay a wee bit more for the blender than you feel comfortable spending, you will feel more obligated to use it. You know—it cost you so much, you have to use it. That can't be a bad motivator. Just sayin'!

3. **Plastic vs. glass:** I used to think that I preferred glass—my Breville was glass—but glass containers can actually be very heavy and break easily. I love the BPA-free polycarbonate plastic that the Vitamix uses, which is also environment friendly. It is easy to wash either manually or with the dishwasher, and it is light. You don't have to be a bodybuilder to lift it out and move it to the counter! So check the blender specification, read up on the quality of the plastic used, and make sure it is dishwasher-safe.

4. **Variable speed settings on the motor:** You ideally want control in the process of making your blends. Variable speed allows you to start on a slower speed, work your way up when your ingredients are mushy, and then bring the speed back down before you finish it. The on/off blenders don't give you any versatility, and therefore zero control. You want different speed settings. This is different from the various settings like "blend," "frothy," "liquefy," and "ice crush," which are more marketing terms than functional terms. Essentially, you want to control the speed at which the blades turn. The Vitamix allows you to go from low to high with many stops along the way. A high-powered machine also allows you to throw everything at once into the blender instead of in stages because you have more control over the blending process.

5. **A tamper to move the ingredients during blending process:** The tamper is the genius part of the Vitamix. Even high-powered machines like the Vitamix need help. The tamper is what you use to help move the food around to make blending easier for your blender. Much, much easier. With my old Breville, I'd have to turn everything off, get a big spoon, swirl things around in the hopes that I got ingredients repositioned well enough, take out the spoon, put the lid back on, and start again. This process would repeat about three to five times for each smoothie. That factor alone would have sealed the deal for me with the Vitamix back then!

If you have your mind set on starting out with a simpler and cheaper blender—and I define cheap as anything under $100—then beware that it won't stand the test of time and frequent pace that you put it through, and you will likely be replacing it soon. If you just want to dabble your toes into the smoothie world, then that's a good place to start. In fact, go with the Nutri or Magic bullets, which are very reasonably priced. I personally loved using them when I was visiting my in-laws. Just beware that cheap may save you money, but it may also frustrate you to the point that you may lose interest in the whole thing. I wouldn't want that to happen to you!

What about using your food processor instead of a blender?

I'm afraid this does not work. You need a proper blender. The food processor is not made in the right shape, lacks the right blades, has neither the motor nor the capacity, and is not equipped to handle liquids well. The food processor blades are made for cutting, slicing, dicing, chopping, and whipping up a mean pesto or homemade hummus. It is not made to break down frozen chunks of fruit or ice the way a proper blender is. If you want to make a decent smoothie on a regular basis, then investing in a blender is the way to go.

Katherine Natalia

Favorite Recipe: Key Lime Pie Green Thickie

2 cups dairy-free milk
2 bananas, frozen
2 tbsp sunflower seeds
¼ cup pitted dates
1 cup spinach, tightly packed, or 2 cups loosely packed (or any other mild greens)
1 cup oats
2–4 limes, just the juice and zest (this tastes amazing with 4 limes, but it's still nice with just 2 limes)
½ teaspoon of vanilla extract

Katherine Natalia is the founder of GreenThickies.com.. Green Thickies are a filling green smoothie containing fruit, greens, carbs, and nuts or seeds. They are designed for busy people so they can get their nutrients and fill themselves up. She invented Green Thickies after having her baby and not having enough time to drink her green smoothies and eat her oatmeal every morning. So she combined the two meals together to make a Green Thickie. Now her whole family enjoys them. Katherine healed herself of Chronic Fatigue Syndrome and many other health problems by changing her diet to a plant-based diet with a large proportion of raw food over three years ago. Katherine also lost fifty-six pounds in the process of healing her body. She is mother to a one-year-old girl with another baby on the way, and lives in Scotland with her husband and daughter. Katherine is passionate about helping people recover their health and reach their ideal weight.

How to Best Shop, Wash, Store, and Plan Ahead for Your Smoothies

If I'd known I was going to live so long, I'd have taken better care of myself.
~Leon Eldred

....

The Shopping

Should you buy organic? Should you buy local? Only when possible. Sure, organically grown food is better for your body than the non-organic version, because it has far less exposure to pesticides and it tastes better. You can also grow your own fruits, vegetables, and greens, but that isn't always practical or budget-friendly. I am not dogmatic about buying *only* organic or local for myself. I do prefer organic, sure, but if I have to choose, I first get my leafy greens organic, then my celery, carrots, berries, lemons, and apples, in that order.

As much as I support the idea of local and organic, I follow it only when my budget and circumstances allow. So do what works for you. Anything that makes this smoothie journey prohibitively expensive or inaccessible is not something you should worry about, because healthy smoothies should be within your reach, no matter what. Believe that!

If you can't buy organic, then buy the freshest fruit and vegetable that you can wherever you find them. Buy what is available in season, as it is always more affordable, and get in the habit of freezing your fruit so it lasts longer and never has a chance to go bad sitting in the fridge, waiting to be eaten. We spend so much time debating the price of our produce, but don't realize how much money we waste by letting it go bad before we use it up! It is literally painful for me to throw away any fruit or vegetable because I didn't plan better in advance. So take heart! If you use every bite of what you buy, you are ahead of the game, no matter what you paid for it!

The Washing

How to thoroughly wash your fruits and vegetables and greens:

- Wash your hands with hot soapy water first.
- Do not ever wash produce with soaps or detergents.
- Use clean, cold water to wash your produce.
- For produce with a thick skin, use a vegetable brush to help wash away skin-surface microbes.
- Produce with a lot of nooks and crannies like cauliflower, broccoli, or lettuce should be soaked for a couple of minutes in clean, cold water.
- Fragile fruits like berries should not be soaked in water. Put them in a colander and run low-pressure cold water through them, or use a water spray.
- Wash the leafy greens by separating leaves from the root (if applicable) and soaking them in a bowl of cool water for a few minutes. Drain the greens using a strainer or colander and repeat this process a few times until all traces of mud and dirt are completely removed.
- Another technique is to presoak greens for five minutes in a mixture of vinegar and water (½ cup white vinegar per two cups water), then follow with a clean water rinse. This has been shown to reduce bacterial contamination, but it may slightly alter texture and taste.
- Drain leafy greens with a clean strainer or colander, then dry with a clean towel or a salad spinner. Wash your salad spinner after every use.
- After washing, dry your fruit and veggies with a clean paper towel. This can remove even more bacteria.
- You do not need to rewash packaged products labeled "ready-to-eat," "washed," or "triple washed."
- Do not purchase cut produce that is not refrigerated.
- Refrigerate your produce immediately after washing and drying. Don't let it sit out at room temperature long if you won't be using the ingredients immediately.

The Storing

Never store your leafy greens in the wet plastic bags you buy them in. The moisture shortens the shelf life of your vegetables fast. Take the time to go through the washing process we talked about. If you are in a hurry, then at the very least take time to remove your produce from the wet bags, dry them with a paper or regular towel, and transfer

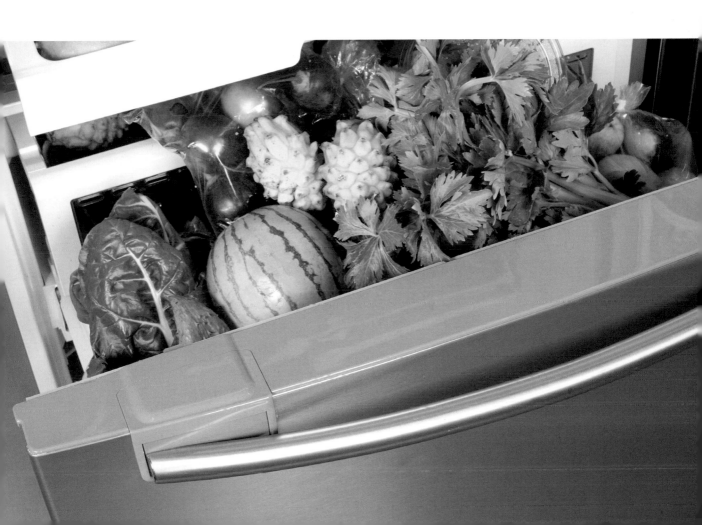

to a plastic container with a lid. You can keep all your leafy greens in clear plastic tubs or zip-top bags in the refrigerator. Add a strip of paper towel or a dry cloth inside the container to absorb excess moisture and condensation.

If you are feeling super organized, add a date of purchase to the container or bag you store it in. Your greens and soft fruits, such as berries, will last you anywhere from three to six days. The denser fruits and vegetables can go a week to ten days. The drier and more moisture-free you can keep your greens, the longer they will last.

The Preparing

So how long does it take to make a smoothie? It depends on the complexity of the recipe. On average, if I have done zero preparation, if nothing is washed or peeled or cut up or prepared, from the minute I walk into my kitchen to when I walk out with a smoothie in hand and the clean Vitamix back on the counter, it takes me between twelve and fifteen minutes if I am leisurely about it, and seven to ten minutes if I am in a mad rush.

Six Tips to Expedite Your Smoothie Making Process for Busy Days

If you don't have that much time in the mornings, you can take a few steps to prepare in advance. Time is of the essence, and when it comes to eating and nourishing our bodies, we always shortchange ourselves. Well, these tips are going to put our bodies and our health first without asking for hours of our time. Follow these tips to expedite your smoothie-making process:

1. **Create a smoothie station in your kitchen**: The more visible your smoothie stuff, the more likely you are to grab it and use it. Put all your tools—cutting board, knife, any containers—and your non-refrigerated foods (like superfoods, dried fruit, nuts, nut butters, and powders) on that station.

2. **Plan your week's recipes ahead of time**: Get out your food journal and plan out your smoothie recipes for the next seven days. Pick recipes that have common fruits and vegetables while also rotating some of your greens. Do your shopping for everything on the weekend.

3. **Organize your smoothie bags**: Get yourself a large box of resealable zip-top bags. For each recipe, go to your fridge, grab all the greens and vegetables the recipe calls for, and put them in a pile on your kitchen counter. Then do the same for fruits. If using frozen fruit, just get the serving size you need and put it in a mason jar, then fill it up with all the greens, veggies, nuts, seeds, or whatever else the recipe calls for. Do not add any liquid to the jar. Put the lid on and store in the fridge. If you are making more than one recipe, make a note of recipes on the jars.

4. **Pour the liquid base in the blender container in advance**: Measure out the liquid base—filtered water or nut milk—into your blender and ideally store it in the refrigerator until ready to make your smoothie. That way you don't have to wash an extra container, and you'll have your liquid ready to go without the need to pour and measure.

5. **Grab, blend, and go**: In the morning or whenever you are ready to make your smoothie in a hurry, just grab your mason jar and dump it into your blender. Your greens will go in first, then your soft fruit, which is mostly defrosted. If your smoothie isn't cold enough, throw a couple of ice cubes in. Then add your smoothie base, blend it up, pour everything back into your smoothie jar, get a straw, and you're done.

6. **Fill your blender with water**: If dashing out the door, just fill your dirty blender with water and soap and let it soak until you wash it later.

Tips on Freezing Your Fruits

So many people spend their health gaining wealth, and then have to spend their wealth to regain their health.
~A.J. Reb Materi

Freezing your own fruit is one of the most fun, economical, and smart things you can do to make your smoothie habit a total breeze. Let's learn how to do this—there's a wee bit more to it than just putting your fruit in a bag and throwing it in the freezer.

Freezing is not for all fruits, sadly. The fruits that you always want to use fresh are apples, oranges, tangerines, grapefruits, lemons, limes, grapes, and pears.

Freezing helps you have out of season fruits all year round. Frozen fruit helps you skip ice and get both the cold and the fruit in one shot. Frozen fruit also gives your smoothie a smooth, creamy texture. And most of all, frozen fruit helps you overcome the short shelf life of fresh fruit. You can extend that shelf life to months—thank you, freezer technology—and never waste a single fruit that might have perished before you got around to using it.

A few guidelines about freezing your fruit: First, don't ever mix fruit. Give each fruit its own dedicated zip-top bag. Bananas get their own bag, and each berry type also gets its own. You may only need blueberries for one recipe, and you don't want to have to separate out one frozen berry from another. Organization is key here. Also, this way you can reuse the same zip-top bag for the same fruit later. Don't use plastic containers in the freezer. The fruit gets stuck to the sides of the container and it takes up way more room than it needs.

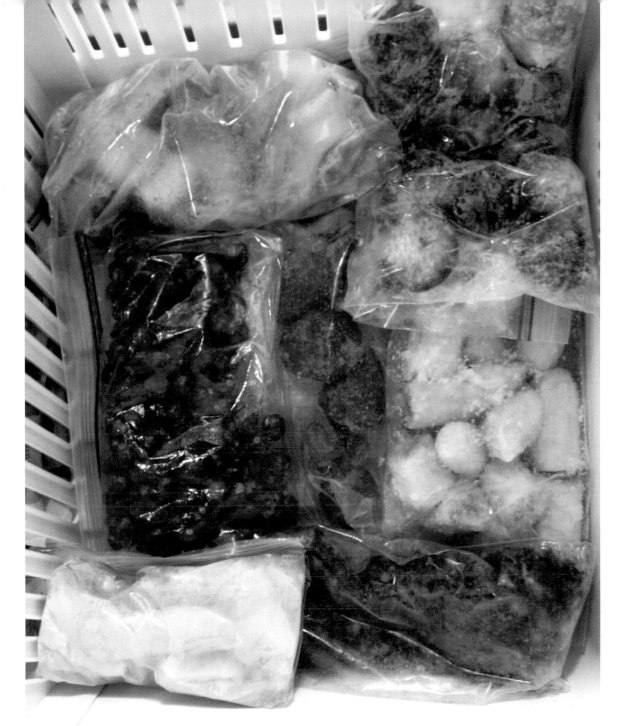

Second, label your zip-top bags using a sharpie. It may sound like overkill, but it's worth it. Take two minutes to write the fruit name and date you started freezing. It helps you sort things out so you use your oldest fruit first. You can keep fruit frozen for months, but I try to use up my frozen fruit in three to six months at most.

Which fruits you should freeze:

Avocado: I love adding frozen avocado as a low-sugar substitute for banana. All the creaminess, and none of the sugar. Plus you get a good dose of healthy fats. Avocados freeze very nicely. First wash your avocado and use a sharp knife to cut it in half (one side will have the pit). Then cut the half into another half, and the pit should come out easily, or you can use a sharp knife when you have the half with the pit, and stick it into the pit to grab it with the knife. Then you can slice off the peel from the half or the quarter avocado. Try to keep that size so you can measure easily. Throw away the skin and just freeze the meat chunks.

Banana: Use only ripe bananas. Peel them first, then use a knife to cut them in halves. That way you can easily measure them when you grab them later. If you think you might get creative and not use one half or one whole banana, then have another zip lock bag with small banana chunks to experiment with.

Berries: Berries have a very short fridge life, so freezing them is such a boon. You can freeze all kinds of berries—my favorites are blueberries, strawberries, blackberries, rasp-berries, and cranberries. Wash your berries well. Run them through lukewarm water for a few minutes using a colander, then dry them with a paper towel before freezing them. Remove the leaves from strawberries and cut them in half with a knife if they are a large size. You may want just a little bit in your smoothie!

Fig: Frozen figs are my top choice for smoothies. I prefer purple figs to the light green ones. They are especially heavenly when you add them to a recipe with soaked gluten-

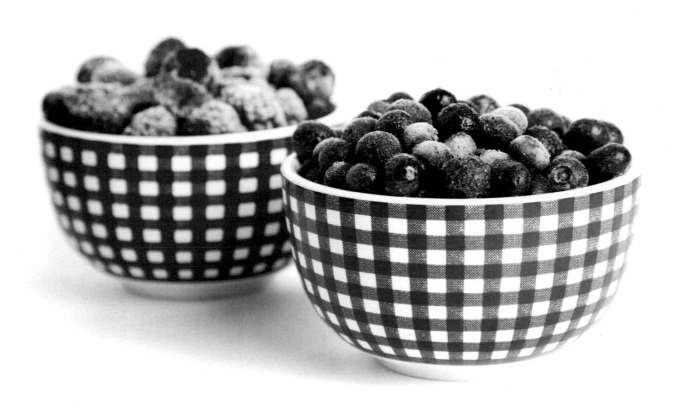

free oats and almond milk. When blended, frozen figs resemble an explosion of purple and pink rainbows. Sadly, figs are hard to find year-round. They come around during the summer months only. Before freezing your figs, wash them thoroughly and cut out the stem. Freeze whole or cut in half. You'll never look back!

Kiwi: Kiwi is another favorite in smoothies. It is not on my top choice list, but it is a delicious fruit and to its credit, it has more vitamin C than a whole orange. Kiwi also freezes nicely. I peel it before freezing it and cut it in halves so it's easy to measure. It's a nice green color that can preserve the color of a green smoothie!

Mango: Fresh mango is delicious, but so is frozen mango. You can freeze your ripe mangos. Either peel them first and cut out small chunks around the core. Or simply cut into halves and use a spoon to scrape out the meat. Put the mango chunks in a zip-top bag in your freezer.

Peach: Peaches freeze very nicely. You do not need to peel the peach, so be sure to wash it well. Then just cut out chunks, throw away the core, and freeze them in a zip-top bag. Peaches do not add as much creaminess as a mango or banana to your smoothie, but it is a nice delicious fruit.

Pineapple: Wash, then peel your pineapple. Be careful not to cut yourself. Chop out the middle hard core section and cut the meats into wedges. Some people prefer to use the core, but it's much too hard to break down if you do not have a high-powered blender, and even though I do, I still don't use it. My rule is simple: If I can't eat it in its fresh state, I don't freeze it! Also try to remove the skin as much as possible. If you have a little bit of the 'eye' left, don't worry, it'll break down. Then put it in your zip-top bag and store it in your freezer.

Pomegranate: Pomegranate is expensive, and you don't want a single seed of this lovely jewel to go to waste, so after de-seeding and washing, you can store them in a zip-top bag in your freezer for up to six months.

THE HEALTHY SMOOTHIE BIBLE

When and Why to Forgo the Ice

One of my tips to enhance the taste of your smoothie is to not use ice, or at least limit the use of ice to an absolute minimum. I suggest you use frozen fruit instead. You can either buy frozen fruit or freeze your own. This way, you get the fruit and the coldness factor in one fell swoop and you pack in so much more flavor.

Fresh fruit tastes better than frozen fruit in smoothies, but frozen fruit lasts longer and you don't have to worry about them perishing three days after purchase. Plus, they require no cleaning, rinsing, or cutting. They are ready to go.

You will notice that a few of the recipes in this book have ice as ingredients—those are probably the ones my husband contributed (only half kidding). It is only when the other ingredients are not cold enough that you need the ice, although it does help thicken the smoothie. Just know that if you have enough frozen fruit in your smoothie, you won't need the ice. Or better yet, use "flavored ice" by pouring your favorite almond milk, hemp milk, or fresh-squeezed orange or carrot juice in an ice cube tray, freeze, and throw the cubes in your smoothie to make it colder.

The most common fruits that you can buy in frozen form are your berries—blueberries, strawberries, raspberries, blackberries, and cranberries—as well as mangos and peaches.

The fruits that you can freeze on your own are avocados, bananas, figs, grapes, pineapple, and kiwis. Of these, I have to admit that frozen figs are my greatest discovery.

Soaking Your Nuts, Seeds, and Oats

While growing up in Iran, I remember that we always had a bowl of nuts soaking in cold water in our refrigerator. I could hardly wait until my mom served them, along with a plate of greens, olives, and goat cheese, a traditional Persian appetizer. The almonds and walnuts were succulent!

One terrific reason to soak your nuts is that many nuts, especially walnuts and almonds, have a much more appealing taste after they are soaked and rinsed properly. As you will see if you try it yourself, after as little as twenty minutes, the soak water turns brown. After a couple hours, a lot of the dust and residue from the skins are released into the water, and the nut emerges with a smoother and much more palatable flavor.

Soaked walnuts lose their astringent taste and become almost sweeter. This is because when soaking walnuts, the tannins are rinsed away, leaving behind a softer, more buttery nut. It is also easier to bite and chew, as it becomes softer while still remaining crunchy.

The best nuts for soaking are almonds, walnuts, peanuts, Brazil nuts, cashews, macadamia nuts, and pecans. There's no need to soak your pistachios or pine nuts. This same soaking process applies to seeds like sunflower seeds, pumpkin seeds, flaxseeds, and sesame seeds, which yields cleaner, better-tasting seeds for your smoothies.

Note that you want to opt for raw nuts, rather than roasted or salted nuts, when you shop. Raw nuts have the most nutrients and natural form for your body and health.

Four-Step Process to Soaking Your Nuts:

1. Put one cup of (de-shelled) nuts with two cups of water in a bowl.
2. Store in the refrigerator for two hours. If pressed for time, do as little as twenty minutes instead of skipping the soaking altogether.

3. Drain and rinse nuts with water if you need to use them immediately. If you want to store them longer, change the water and soak for another four to six hours.
4. Rinse a second time. Dry nuts by wrapping and pressing them gently in a towel. Always discard the brown soak water from nuts and seeds; do not drink it or use it in a recipe.

Store nuts in a closed glass container in the fridge for use in your smoothies. Avoid using plastic if possible.

Soaking also helps soften the hard coating of oats. You do not need to soak and rinse the oats in water, however. This is slightly different.

Three-Step Process to Soaking Your Oats:

1. Use one cup of your base, such as filtered water or any non-dairy milk, to soak ½ cup of oats the night before you need your smoothie, or four hours in advance if preparing in the middle of the day.
2. Cover the mixture with plastic wrap or put in a closed container in the refrigerator.
3. Pour into your blender when ready to make your smoothie.

If you don't get a chance to soak your oats in advance and are in a hurry and determined to make that recipe with oats, worry not! Just put the oats in the blender first by themselves without any liquid and run the blender for thirty seconds to "powderize" them, as my hubby says. Then proceed with the rest of your ingredients. Enjoy!

Some of the benefits of soaking nuts and seeds is the increased enzyme activity, as well as the ease of absorption of these nuts by your digestive system. When you soak them, you are activating their natural sprouting process, which increases their nutritional profile greatly.

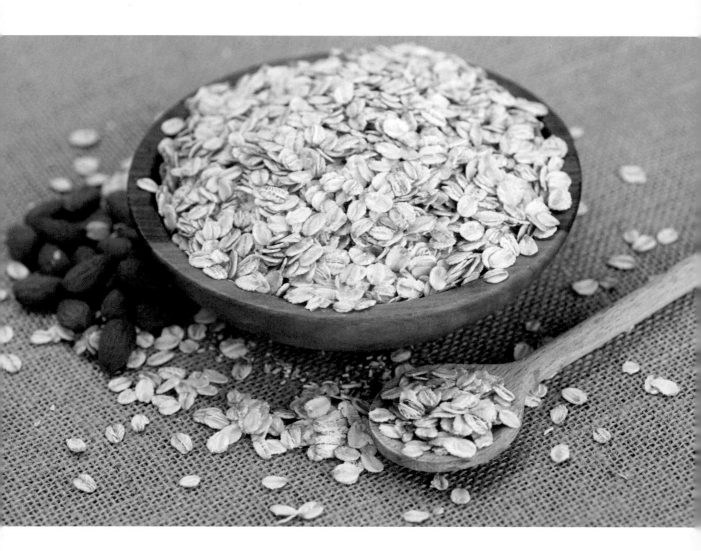

THE HEALTHY SMOOTHIE BIBLE

Steps to Make Your Smoothie

Health is not valued until sickness comes.
~Thomas Fuller

You now have everything you need to start making your smoothie. The instructions are simple:

1. You throw your ingredients into your blender in a sensible order and with the matching liquid base.
2. You blend to your desired consistency. You stop. You pour. You enjoy!

That's the essence of making smoothies when things go smoothly (no pun intended), and the good news is that it happens that way most of the time. But just to give you more power behind making the perfect smoothie, here are a few more tips:

Your smoothie can take on any consistency you desire. Always go for thick first, because you can always thin it with water, but not necessarily the other way around. Remember, depending on whether your blender is a high-powered blender or a regular one, you may use a different amount of liquid to achieve the same consistency. So adjust your actual liquid base based on that factor.

If you get a chunk of frozen fruit just circling the blender without getting caught in the blade, you're probably blending too fast. Slow down or pulse a few times and your blender will break it down afterward.

If you've added your whole base and the blender is still having trouble, use the tamper (if you have one) while blending to move things around, or stop the blender and use a long wooden spoon to move things. Another option is to add ½ to ¾ cup of water to any smoothie, which should get everything moving again.

If you want to be very systematic about it, always add your liquid base first so that you can measure it with the blender's readings. Then add your soft fruit, greens, nuts, and lastly add frozen fruit.

How long should you blend for? The short answer is, until you get the desired consistency, but the more efficient you are, the better. Your ideal blending time is anywhere from one minute to ninety seconds. Most high-powered blenders can meet this time without a problem. With smaller, less powerful blenders, you may have to help the blender more to get things going, and thus the whole thing may take longer. Be patient. You will get the hang of your blender soon.

Try not to blend for more than two minutes at most, or you risk oxidation and nutrient loss. This is where a high-powered blender like the Vitamix or Blendtec is such a boon. It takes about half the time to give you that professionally done, smooth, silky drink!

Tasting the Smoothie and Salvaging a Smoothie Gone Wrong

When blending has ended, dip in a spoon to taste your smoothie before serving it up. If you love it, then bon appetit. If not, before you dump it out in the sink as a loss, let's see if we can salvage it together.

Is it too thick? Then use water or more of your base to thin it out. The easiest problem to fix!

Is it too thin? You can add thickeners like banana, avocado, coconut, or more of whatever is already in the smoothie.

Is it not cold enough? Add ice, or if it is also not sweet enough or balanced with enough fruity flavor, use more of your frozen fruit.

Is it bitter or not sweet enough? Add more of the same fruit to balance the sweetness, or add one or two pitted dates.

Is it too sweet? You can always add more water, if that's your liquid base, to dilute the sweetness. You can also add a handful of mild greens, like spinach, to cut down the sweetness.

Is it too bland? Then add some cinnamon, nutmeg, pumpkin spice, or vanilla extract to give it more flavor. If it's a savory smoothie, spice it up with cayenne pepper, sea salt, hot spices, or garlic.

How Much to Drink, and How Much is Too Much?

On an average day, I drink between sixteen to twenty-eight ounces of green and/or non-green healthy smoothie. It makes up for at least one of my meals and ideally covers me for all my snacks. Then I am ready to chew something for the remaining meal(s). Chewing is extremely important, and it's one of the reasons why you should not just go with an all-smoothie diet, unless you take up some jaw-strengthening exercises!

How much you drink is up to you, and at first, drink only however much you like. If it's just a cup, then that's that. You can build up as you find your favorite recipes and ways of making your smoothie. If you can drink sixteen ounces of smoothie on a relatively regular schedule, about four or five times a week, you are doing spectacularly!

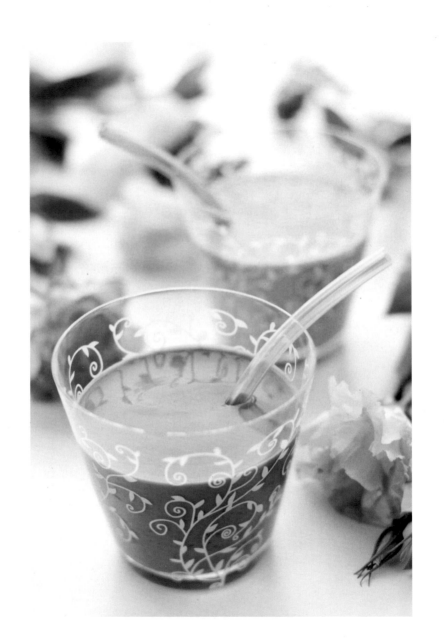

Getting the Right Texture for Your Smoothie

The texture of your smoothie is a function of three things: the ingredients, the type of blender, and the length of time you blend. Remember, you don't always want to have a smooth-textured recipe.

You may want to have a more chewy result one day, a more hydrating one another day, or sometimes a thick smoothie. The "smoothifiers", if I may use that word, are the binding elements—your avocados, bananas, mangoes, and coconut meat are on top of that list. You can always re-blend if you have chunks that are not entirely blended in.

How Best to Clean Your Blender

The easiest and fastest way to clean your blender is to give it a quick rinse with warm water immediately after use, along with some dishwashing soap. Nothing has half a chance to stick to the walls, and no need to scrub at all. If you are in a hurry, then fill your blender with water and leave it in the sink until you are ready to wash it.

You can also self-wash the blender! Fill your blender ¾ of a cup full with warm water and soap and give it a nice scrub on the insides. Place it back on your blender stand and turn the machine on for thirty seconds: it's like a mini-dishwasher at work. Of all my blenders, the Vitamix is the easiest to wash. It helps tremendously that it's not made of glass, which is heavy and needs to be handled gently.

To Store or Not Store Your Smoothie?

A healthy body is the guest-chamber of the soul; a sick, its prison.
~Francis Bacon

You can technically store smoothies up to a day or two in the fridge. Here are a few things to know first.

First, be aware that smoothies tend to lose their original flavor and begin to taste different after being stored. Even if you store them for only two or three hours, you will taste a different drink than the one you had fresh out of the blender. For this reason alone, I don't really like storing my smoothies more than an hour max, and sometimes that's just to chill a smoothie that I did not want to make with ice or frozen ingredients.

The other change you will notice after storing the smoothie is a different texture and color. Some of the fruits and vegetables begin to oxidize, and you will notice a new layer on the very top of the smoothie. You can always just spoon that off or mix it in and forget you ever saw it, but yes, it's totally fine to eat it.

The change that you won't notice is the lower nutritional potency. Naturally, when things are fresh, they have the highest amount of vitamins and minerals, but with storage, some of that dissipates. It is still good for you on the nutrition scale, but less so than its fresh version. The less time that passes between the end of blending and the smoothie reaching your body, the better!

If you are definitely going to store your smoothie, then follow these tips below:

1. Always use glass containers rather than plastic. Glass keeps the taste of the smoothie intact, whereas plastic sometimes adds its own, shall we say, "flavor"? Make sure

your glass container is completely airtight. Use containers that have airtight bail and seal closures to hermetically seal out air and moisture. Glass mason jars with BPA-free plastic reusable lids are perfect and very affordable. One of my all-time favorites is the Bormioli Rocco Fido brand, which you can get on Amazon.

2. Fill the container to the very top. This way you prevent any air from being trapped in the container, because air will oxidize the nutrients in your smoothie, which lowers the nutritional content.

3. Seal your container tightly and store in the refrigerator for ideally no more than twenty-four hours.

4. If you want to make your smoothie last even longer, squeeze a little fresh lemon or lime juice over it before you store it. The extra vitamin C will also help prevent oxidation.

Should you freeze your smoothies? I have never frozen mine. If you are curious, pour your smoothie into your ice tray and freeze a couple of cubes of it. Then defrost and see if you like the taste. I do want to encourage you to take the time to make *fresh* smoothies, if only to get your greens at their freshest. Freezing should be a very last resort.

As always, you make the call, so if you decide to store, experiment to see if it works. Taste your smoothie after a couple of hours and see if you notice much difference. Taste it after a day to see if it's any different. I personally prefer not to store if I can help it, but sometimes, opening the fridge and finding that leftover smoothie solves all my otherwise worse impulse snacking decisions!

Rule of thumb: Fresh is best, and it tastes the greatest. I say store as a last resort, and no more than a few hours at that. Smoothies are not the type of food that you can prepare in advance, so focus on how you can expedite the prep process instead.

Jen Hansard and Jadah Sellner

Favorite Recipe: Citrus Breeze

2 cups spinach
1½ cups filtered water
½ cup frozen mango
½ cup fresh or frozen pineapple
2 navel oranges, peeled
1 frozen or fresh banana

Jen and Jadah are two friends on a mission to spread the love of green smoothies. They have changed the lives of over 300,000 people through their free Thirty-Day Green Smoothie Challenge at simplegreensmoothies.com. They are both moms to young children and know how exhausting and busy life can be. In 2011, they decided to embark on a green smoothie journey, even though they live far from each other (Jadah lives in California and Jen lives in Florida). Together, they have lost weight, gained more energy, and nourished their children without so much as a fuss! It all started with a simple green smoothie. These plant-powered green drinks are packed full of leafy greens, fresh fruits, and hydrating liquids that keep you nourished and your cravings at bay for hours. By introducing more leafy greens into your diet, you will reap the benefits of phytonutrients, antioxidants, and essential vitamins and minerals.

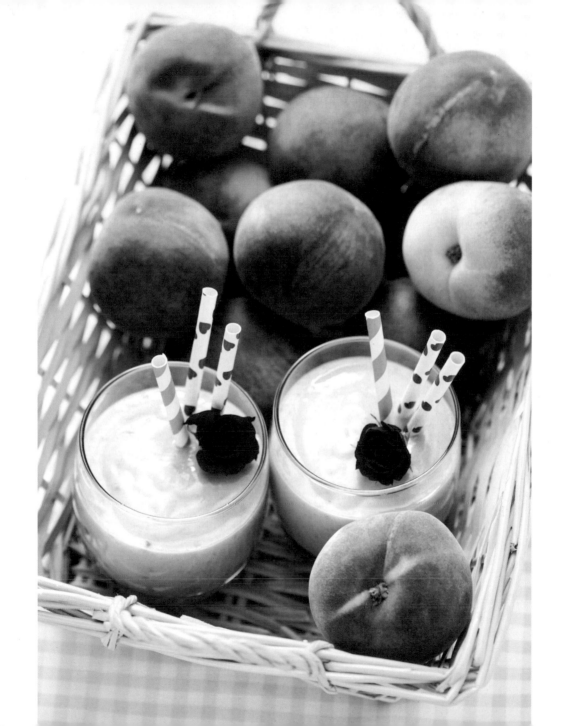

108 Delectable Healthy Smoothie Recipes

Every human being is the author of his own health or disease.
~**Buddha**

We have at last arrived at our sweet spot: the recipe section. Are you ready? A ton of creativity and experimentation, infused with a lot of heart and soul, went into these recipes. I wanted to keep them simple, but also move beyond the strawberry-banana-spinach smoothie that is not very interesting after the tenth time you make it. And that's my first word of advice: Don't get stuck with the same one or two recipes. Switch it up, explore, play with new tastes, get new types of greens, and use fruit that you have not bought or tasted before. You will love finding new favorites, and your body will thank you for the richness of nutrition.

You will notice that we have 108 recipes here, not counting our featured recipes from contributors. I selected 108 because it is a sacred number in many world faiths, including yoga, which has been a constant healing force in my life. Because our theme here in this smoothie path is healing, I wanted to add a special emphasis on healing thoughts and deeds to remind you of that.

Regarding the recipes, I assure you that I've personally made and tasted every single recipe at least once, and on average, two to three times. I tried—and sometimes succeeded—to get my husband to do a taste-test for me. I subjected some of my good friends to the same fun test.

If you are the type of person who loves to follow a recipe like a baker—in other words, extremely exact and measuring down to teaspoons and ounces—then please relax. Smoothie-making is not a science. These recipes are as exact as it made sense to be, and not any more. There is room to play and to explore, and your results may vary from mine depending on your measurement units and produce size and density.

Making smoothies is an exercise beyond following a recipe. It's one with playing and giving yourself the permission to be free and have fun. With that said, let's jump into our sweet recipes.

About the 108 Smoothie Recipes

The cure of the part should not be attempted without the cure of the whole.
~Plato

All the recipes in this book are vegan. There are no dairy or other animal products in any of the recipes in the Healthy Smoothie Recipes section. You may, however, find dairy in the contributor recipes at the end of each chapter, with an explanation of that recipe.

All of the recipes are also gluten-free, except where noted otherwise. Gluten is known to cause anywhere from mild sensitivity to extreme pain and other health problems, and since eating a relatively low-gluten diet, I feel so much better. One thing I can tell you if you are indifferent about gluten—you won't miss it when you remove it from your diet.

A note to the raw foodie lovers among you: Every recipe can also be made raw. The nuts used in these recipes are all unroasted and unprocessed. The nut milks can be raw when they are homemade. I have used mostly high-quality brands of packaged nut milks. See more in the "Using Non-Dairy Milks as a Base" section about nut milks.

As far as nut butters go, again if they are made at home, they can be made raw. Whole Foods and several similar health food stores let you make your own nut butters using their machines. Just make sure the nuts are raw and unroasted. My nut butter of choice is almond butter, but I do love the taste of peanut butter and have included it in some recipes. Both almond butter and peanut butter are good sources of protein and dietary fiber.

If you want to use peanut butter, make sure you are not getting overly processed peanut butter in jars. Either make it at home or use the machines at the store to make it right there. Almond butter is more expensive and not as widely available commercially. As with peanut butter, either make yours at home or fresh in the store using their machines. I store homemade or fresh nut butters for up to two weeks. If you buy it in a jar, use a top brand and look at the ingredients section for words such as no preservatives and additives or partially hydrogenated oils (trans fats!), or any added sugars. The only listing on the ingredients should be nuts and salt, unless you are choosing the unsalted variety, which is even better.

One of the main reasons I have opted for almond butter over peanut butter in the majority of those recipes including nut butters is the high allergy rates to peanut butter. If you have any allergies to peanuts, take care to stay far away from them. I have not tried cashew butter, but you can just as easily substitute it in.

If you want to get adventurous, go for exotic nut butters like macadamia butter, hazelnut butter, walnut butter, or pistachio butter. Just keep in mind that it might get expensive and they are not as readily available for regular use.

Speaking of exotic, I have used easy-to-find, simple ingredients in the majority of these recipes. I wanted to make them accessible to you no matter where you live. There are also alternatives and replacement options if you can't find a particular green or fruit in your part of the world. Almost all recipes are adaptable to what you have available at home or in your hometown grocery shop. My goal was sneaky: I wanted to remove all excuses so you get down to it and make healthy smoothies a part of your lifestyle.

All nut milks are the unsweetened version unless otherwise specified.

How Best to Go Through the Recipes Section

At first, you can skim over the recipes quickly and check the ingredients to see which ones speak to you. Keep an eye on the tags as you go through them. After skimming, you can use the recipes index at the back of the book to mark your favorites by name for later. You can make recipes based on what you have handy and ready to go in your fridge, or do some pre-planning if you want to go about it in a more organized way.

What I recommend is to start with beginner recipes if you are new to smoothies, and do that for two weeks. Then move to the hidden greens recipes and let your taste buds adjust to the greens, which I promise you will barely taste, if at all. More than anything, let your mind get on board with greens in a fruit smoothie. You can move to super greens in three weeks or less if you are consistent with making smoothies at least five times a week.

Persian-Inspired Ingredients

You will notice that I include some ingredients that are inspired by my culture and background. I am from Iran, the old land of Persia, and we love our fruits and vegetables, our foods and spices. So to honor my culture, I have used some of Persia's favorite ingredients in my recipes. These include figs (frozen and fresh), pomegranate, dates, saffron, jasmine rice (it's only one special recipe!), and pistachios.

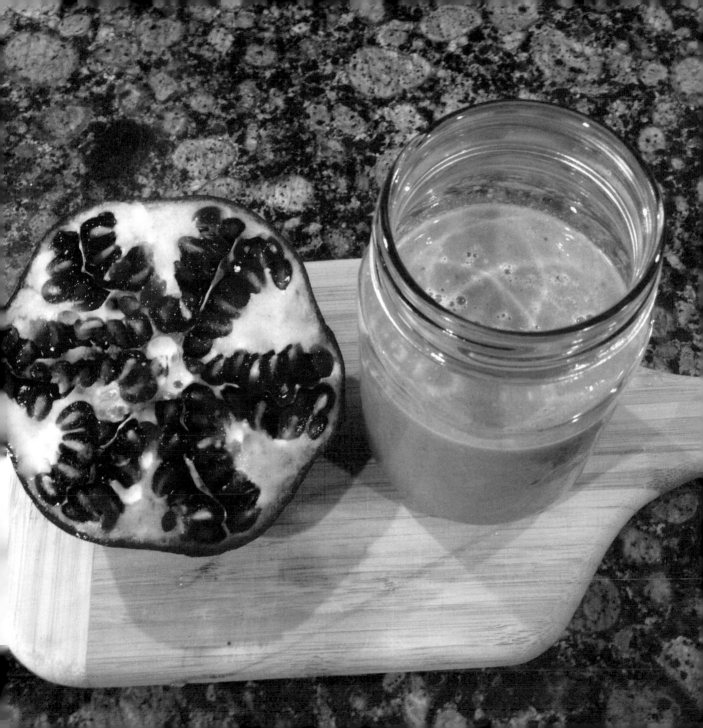

Measurement Units Used in the Recipes

I wanted to keep the measurements simple yet accurate. You will find that unless you measure everything on a scale, it is impossible to get the same exact measures in your smoothie as I would in mine. But here's the thing: You can come close and approximate, and you will be fine. Making smoothies is not as scientific as baking, or else I would not be writing this book. The produce you buy varies and the packaging—or "bunching up" as I like to call it—especially varies. The measurement units are a guideline. Soon, you will not even measure because you will start to eyeball your recipes based on your experience and your expertise.

When I say a cup of greens, it is a well-packed cup. As you know, greens are light and leafy, so you want to press them a little to make sure you fill in the space and make it a nice full and fair cup!

When I say one whole or half a single fruit, it is based on a medium-sized fruit.

And now let's attack the one I got some grief for: a handful. I struggled about whether I should use handful or cup measurements here for the greens, and I stuck with handful. When I say a handful, it is your handful. Whatever you can comfortably grab in your hand, that's it. Whether you grab three more leaves of spinach than me in that handful is not going to affect your taste or your yield significantly. What matters more is that one handful is distinctly different than two handfuls! I also didn't want you to waste time measuring your greens in a cup every time before throwing them into your blender.

In the case of the more bitter greens, you may see unit measurements such as four leaves of dandelion, because they are strong and bitter and a little goes a long way.

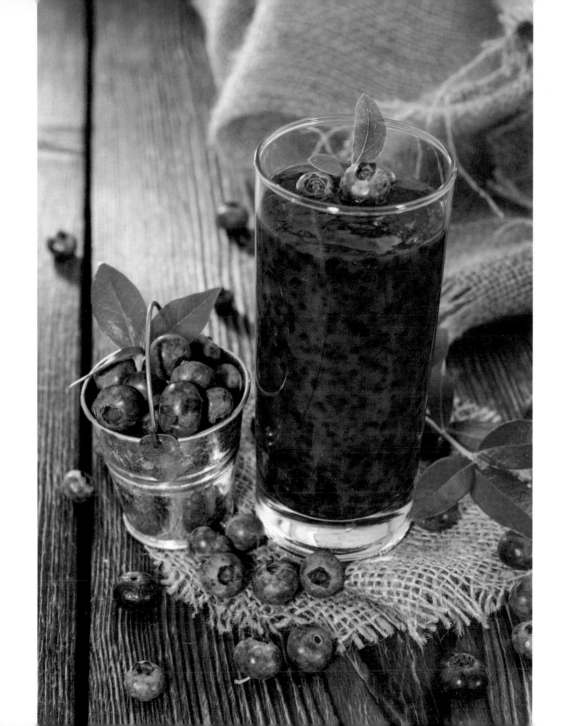

Also, remember that making smoothies is not an exact science. Even the same recipe may yield different results. One time you may be more generous with your greens, and sometimes your apple or pear will vary in size to the previous time. You can't go wrong, and you can salvage most smoothies when you may have put a little too much or too little of something by adjusting after your first blend.

How Much Green is Ideal in Your Smoothie?

To make it super simple for you, you will be fine in most cases with two handfuls of a variety of greens, or the same green, as long as you rotate through different kinds. Over time, your taste buds will change, so you may want to add even more greens or different types of greens. You will not easily overdose on greens, so use as much as you like.

Recipe Yields: How Many Servings?

The measurements in these recipes yield anywhere from two to four cups. They are meant to be between one and two servings. This obviously depends on how much you plan to drink. I define a serving of smoothie as two cups. I like to drink two to four cups of smoothie, or sixteen to thirty-two ounces, for a complete meal or before I am satisfied. I linger over it and drink it over a half-hour period. Another factor to take into account with servings is how thick you make your smoothie. Naturally, a thicker, denser smoothie will fill you up faster with a smaller serving size. I like a thick smoothie when I am hungry and a thin smoothie—for lack of a better word—when I am thirsty and in need of hydration.

Worry-Free Approach to Calories

What? Did I just say that? Why, yes, I did. There is no calorie information on any of the recipes. This book is not about counting your calories and starving yourself on a daily allotment of 850 calories. Besides, depending on your rate of metabolism, you may be able to put away twice as much in smoothie calories than my husband or I could. Calories can be a good indicator of how much food and fuel comes in a glass of smoothie, but it is not the focus of this book. The focus is to get healthy, fresh, whole foods into your body in a blended form. Drink your smoothies until you are full, then save the rest. Instead of counting calories, focus on listening to your body's cues.

The Adaptable Nutritional Table

I have also left out the nutritional tables. There are a few reasons. Whole fruit and vegetable sizes can vary. The actual type of liquid base you use (i.e., sweetened or unsweetened almond milk) will matter. You may also modify and improve your recipes with optional additions and/or replacements. If you choose to use broccoli instead of cauliflower, or no tomato because you have allergies, then the nutritional tables are rendered useless. But while there are no nutritional tables, you can learn more about the benefits of the fruits, vegetables, greens, and superfoods in the relevant sections.

Smart Recipe Tags

To help you identify which recipes are the best fit for you during a particular situation or day of the week, or even stage of the game in your smoothie journey, I've created seven Smart Recipe Tags for us. You will find these tags next to each recipe. Each recipe has at least one tag, but may have several to help you decide which to make at a glance.

Here's a description for each of the Smart Recipe Tags:

1. **Quick:** This is your quick and dirty smoothie for when you are in a big rush. It's for those mornings when you barely have time for breakfast, or those afternoons when you have five minutes to whip up a healthy snack. These recipes are quick! No peeling. No cutting. No preparation in advance.

2. **Low Fruit:** This is for low-sugar lovers. If you are following a low-carb diet, these recipes are ideal for you. These smoothies contain zero or very little fruit. The overall fructose level is lower than other recipes, yet they are still delicious and tasty.

3. **Beginner:** If you are new to smoothies, you will get the good old familiar tastes with these recipes. I promise these recipes don't have any greens or exotic ingredients, and they are a perfect way to get your feet—or mouth!—wet with smoothies.

4. **Green Lover:** When you are ready for a powerhouse of nutrition from the greens, look for this tag. These recipes are green-heavy, but still contain some fruit and possibly other superfoods to make them delightfully palatable.

5. **Hidden Green:** This tag is when you want to sneak a handful of greens into a smoothie but don't want anyone to know. It's the tricky smoothie for kids and for fooling loved ones who have sworn off a "green" drink. These recipes do not come out green, even though they have a hidden green or two that adds the nutrition without the fuss.

THE HEALTHY SMOOTHIE BIBLE

6. **Meal Replacement:** These smoothies give you a filling and richer smoothie. They usually contain extra proteins, fats, or possibly an extra dose of delicious nutrients that keep you going for hours. They are higher in calories and can replace breakfast, lunch and sometimes even dinner. These are also great smoothies for a post-workout meal.

7. **Detox & Cleanse:** This is for all the smoothies that you can have during a Detox & Cleanse—see the section on the Green Smoothie Detox Regimen. These smoothies only contain water, ice, fresh or frozen fruit, fresh vegetables, and greens. No nuts, nut milks, nut butters, seeds, powders, or superfoods here. Watch out for these ingredients before you add optional additions of recipes tagged with Detox & Cleanse, as tagging is based on the original recipe.

8. **Farnoosh's Signature Gems:** This tag is for my own signature smoothies. Some are influenced by my Persian fruits and spices, and all are unbeatable awesome recipes. These are my true favorites, my staple recipes, and my glowing healers, and they're yours to enjoy!

Smart Recipe Tag	Recipe Numbers
Beginner	1, 4, 5, 6, 7, 8, 16, 20, 21, 22, 23, 24, 25, 27, 29, 31, 33, 34, 37, 38, 39, 40, 41, 42, 43, 44, 47, 48, 50, 56, 58, 61, 62, 63, 64, 65, 67, 68, 69, 75, 81, 88, 91, 94, 98, 99, 100, 102, 107, 108
Quick	1, 5, 7, 8, 9, 11, 14, 19, 24, 29, 30, 32, 36, 38, 42, 45, 46, 47, 51, 53, 54, 55, 59, 60, 65, 66, 67, 69, 75, 88, 93, 94, 95, 96, 98, 100, 101, 105, 107, 108
Detox & Cleanse	1, 3, 5, 9, 10, 11, 15, 16, 17, 19, 35, 46, 49, 51, 53, 57, 66, 70, 73, 74, 76, 80, 83, 84, 85, 89, 91, 93, 96, 97, 99, 101, 102, 104, 107, 108
Meal Replacement	2, 3, 7, 12, 13, 14, 20, 21, 22, 23, 26, 27, 28, 31, 32, 34, 37, 38, 43, 45, 48, 52, 55, 56, 69, 72, 74, 77, 79, 82, 86, 90, 92
Green Lover	2, 9, 10, 15, 17, 25, 30, 35, 36, 46, 49, 53, 54, 57, 59, 60, 70, 71, 72, 73, 74, 76, 80, 83, 84, 89, 96, 97, 101, 104
Farnoosh's Signature Gems	16, 40, 41, 43, 44, 48, 49, 57, 66, 70, 73, 78, 80, 81, 82, 86, 87, 90, 91, 92, 97, 99, 102, 103, 108
Low Fruit	9, 11, 33, 36, 47, 49, 56, 58, 61, 62, 68, 73, 74, 76, 78, 84, 89, 95, 100, 105, 106
Hidden Green	4, 6, 7, 11, 13, 18, 28, 33, 39, 41, 43, 48, 52, 62, 64, 77, 78, 79, 85, 87, 101, 106

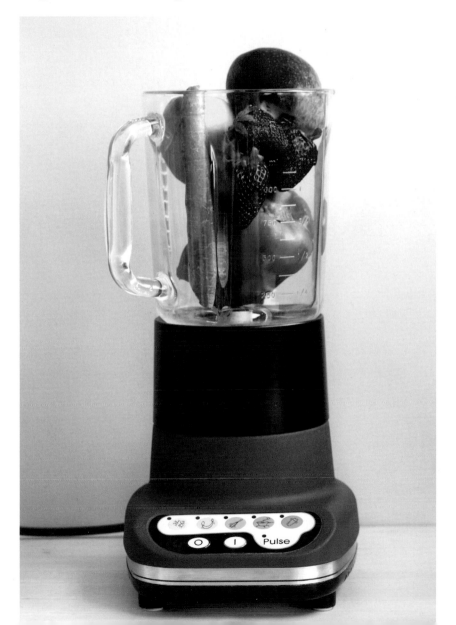

Recipe #1: Green Mango Chill

Tags: Quick, Beginner, Detox & Cleanse

Ingredients:

1 cup filtered water
1 cup frozen mango
1 medium frozen banana
2 cups chopped celery
1 handful of parsley

Replacements:

Cilantro for parsley

Recipe #2: Wake Me Up Green Essence

Tags: Green Lover, Meal Replacement

Ingredients:

A small handful fresh oregano
1 frozen banana
1 handful spinach
2 large leaves of kale, without stem
1 peeled orange
$\frac{1}{3}$ cup soaked walnuts
1 cup filtered water

Replacements:

Spinach for kale

Notes:

Wash and soak walnuts in filtered water overnight. Use in smoothie the next day.

....

Recipe #3: Minty Pineapple Love

Tags: Meal Replacement, Detox & Cleanse

Ingredients:

½ large avocado
1 handful of fresh mint
2 cups fresh Swiss chard, no stem
1 cup frozen pineapple
1 cup filtered water
1 cup ice cubes
Optional additions:
¼ cup soaked walnuts or almonds

Notes:

Wash and soak walnuts or almonds in filtered water overnight. Use in smoothie the next day.

Recipe #4: Nutty Berry Prospect

Tags: Hidden Green, Beginner

Ingredients:

1 large frozen banana
3 large frozen strawberries
½ cup frozen blueberries
2 cups fresh baby spinach
1 cup filtered water
1 tbsp peanut butter

Replacements:

Almond butter for peanut butter

Recipe #5: Green Grape Delight

Tags: Beginner, Quick, Detox & Cleanse

Ingredients:

1 large frozen banana
1 handful of fresh mint
20 fresh white seedless grapes
5–6 leaves romaine lettuce
⅓ large fresh peeled avocado
1 cup filtered water
½ lemon, juice squeezed into the blender
Optional additions:
A small chunk of peeled ginger

Recipe #6: Pineapple Kale Explosion

Tags: Hidden Green, Beginner

Ingredients:

1 large frozen banana
3–4 medium leaves of kale, no stem
1 cup fresh pineapple
1 cup fresh blueberries
1 cup filtered water
¼ cup raw soaked pecans or almonds
Optional additions:
1 handful of fresh mint

Notes:

Wash and soak pecans or almonds in filtered water overnight. Use in smoothie the next day.

Recipe #7: The Celery Nutcase

Tags: Meal Replacement, Beginner, Hidden Green, Quick

Ingredients:

4 large frozen strawberries
1 frozen banana
3 large fresh celery stalks
1 cup frozen mango
1 cup filtered water
1 tbsp almond butter

Recipe #8: Romaine Ginger Potency

Tags: Beginner, Quick

Ingredients:

1 frozen peeled avocado
A small chunk of fresh peeled ginger
1 fresh peeled kiwi
5–6 leaves of romaine lettuce
1 cup coconut milk

Optional addition:
1 tbsp sesame seeds

Replacements:

Spinach for lettuce

Recipe #9: The Kiwi-Parsley Rapture

Tags: Green Lover, Quick, Detox & Cleanse, Low Fruit

Ingredients:

1 frozen peeled avocado
1 handful fresh mint
1 handful fresh spinach
1 handful fresh parsley
1 fresh peeled kiwi
1 cup filtered water

Optional addition:

½ fresh lemon juice squeezed into blender

Recipe #10: Hydrating Chard Potion

Tags: Green Lover, Detox & Cleanse

Ingredients:

2 cups fresh Swiss chard, without stem
1 handful fresh parsley
1 large frozen banana
2 cucumbers, unpeeled
1 medium granny smith apple, de-cored
1 small chunk of ginger
1 cup filtered water

Recipe #11: Love Me Some Kale

Tags: Hidden Green, Quick, Detox & Cleanse, Low Fruit

Ingredients:

2 cups fresh kale, without stem
3 frozen strawberries
¼ cup frozen blueberries
1 frozen peeled avocado
1 cup filtered water

Replacements:

Spinach for kale

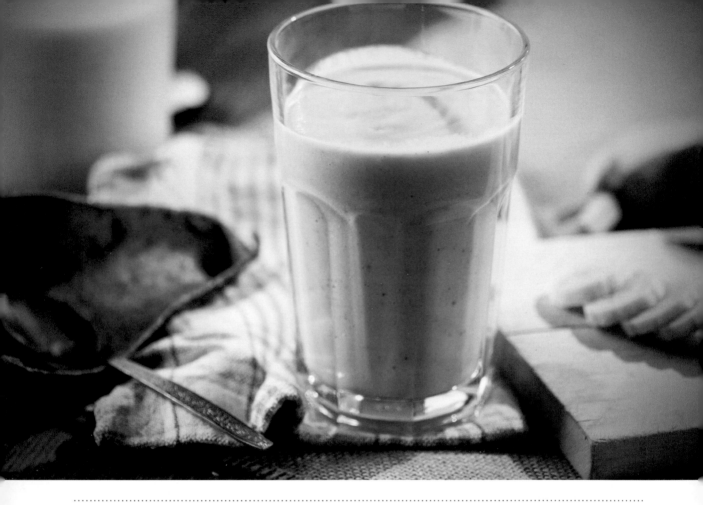

Recipe #12: Creamy Filling Delight

Tags: Meal Replacement

Ingredients:

½ frozen peeled avocado
1 frozen banana

142

1 small cucumber
2 cups fresh romaine lettuce
1 handful of fresh mint
10 soaked walnuts or almonds
1 cup filtered water

Optional additions:

1 small chunk of ginger

Notes:

Wash and soak walnuts or almonds in filtered water overnight. Use in smoothie the next day.

....

Recipe #13: Zesty Berry Morning

Tags: Hidden Green, Meal Replacement

Ingredients:

8–10 blackberries
1 large frozen banana
2 cups fresh spinach
½ cup frozen mango
⅓ cup raw soaked pecans
1 peeled orange
1 cup filtered water

Optional additions:

1 tbsp sesame seeds

Notes:

Soak pecans in filtered water overnight. Use in smoothie the next day.

Recipe #14: Cran-Banana Deluxe

Tags: Quick, Meal Replacement

Ingredients:

1 frozen banana
½ cup fresh cranberries
2 cups fresh spinach
1 tbsp almond butter
1 cup filtered water

Recipe #15: Fruity Festive Sensation

Tags: Green Lover, Detox & Cleanse

Ingredients:

1 medium sweet apple
1 peeled orange
2 cups fresh spinach
1 handful of fresh parsley
1 frozen peeled avocado
1 cup filtered water

Optional additions:

1 small chunk of ginger

Recipe #16: Citrus Superload

Tags: Beginner, Detox & Cleanse, Farnoosh's Signature Gem

Ingredients:

1 cup fresh or frozen pineapple
2 small cucumbers
2 cups fresh spinach
½ frozen peeled avocado
1 orange, peeled
½ lemon juice squeezed into the blender
1 small chunk of ginger
1 cup filtered water

Optional additions:

1 handful of fresh mint

Replacements:

Romaine lettuce for spinach
Lime juice for lemon juice

Recipe #17: My Green Fantasy

Tags: Green Lover, Detox & Cleanse

Ingredients:

1 frozen banana
½ frozen avocado
4–5 leaves of romaine lettuce
1 handful fresh cilantro
1 cup baby spinach
1 cup filtered water

Optional additions:
½ lime, juice squeezed into blender

Replacements:

Romaine lettuce for spinach

Recipe #18: Chia Mango Sunrise

Tags: Hidden Green

Ingredients:

1 tbsp chia seeds
1 tsp sesame seeds
1–1½ frozen banana
½ cup frozen blueberries

½ cup frozen mango
⅓ cup soaked raw almonds
1 cup filtered water

Optional additions:

½ lemon, peeled
A small chunk of ginger

Notes:

Soak almonds in filtered water overnight. Use in smoothie the next day.

....

Recipe #19: Sweet Sexy Cooler

Tags: Quick, Detox & Cleanse

Ingredients:

1 frozen banana
1 cup frozen mango
½ fresh Pink Lady or Golden Delicious apple
1 cup fresh spinach
1 cup fresh fennel, leaves and bulb

Optional additions:

1 small chunk of ginger

Recipe #20: Post-Workout Power Chai Infusion

Tags: Meal Replacement, Beginner

Ingredients:

1 tbsp hemp seeds
1¼ cup coconut milk
1 packet of Amazing Meal Vanilla Chai Infusion (by Amazing Grass)
½ cup frozen blueberries
1 frozen banana
2–3 frozen strawberries
1 tbsp chia seeds or powder

Replacements:

Use your favorite vanilla-flavored meal replacement or protein powder.

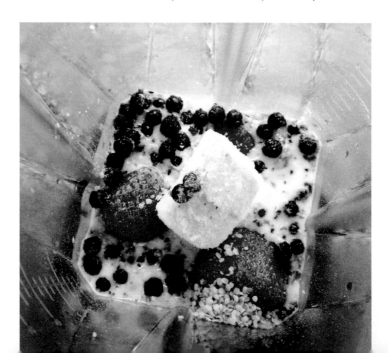

Recipe #21: Chocolate Strawberry Fling

Tags: Meal Replacement, Beginner

Ingredients:

1 frozen banana
1 portion of Amazing Grass Amazing Meal Chocolate Infusion
1 cup frozen strawberries
1 tbsp hemp seeds
1–1¼ cup coconut milk

Optional additions:

1 tsp chia seeds

Replacements:

Use your favorite meal replacement or protein powder instead.

Recipe #22: Sunwarrior Sunday

Tags: Meal Replacement, Beginner

Ingredients:

1 packet of Sunwarrior plant-based chocolate raw protein powder
1 tbsp peanut butter
1 frozen banana
1 cup almond milk

Replacements:

Use your favorite meal replacement or protein powder instead
Use almond butter for peanut butter

....

Recipe #23: Raw Warrior Class

Tags: Meal Replacement, Beginner

Ingredients:

1 scoop Raw Warrior Rice Protein Powder
2 cups fresh spinach
1 frozen banana
1 peeled orange
1 cup filtered water

Optional additions:

1 tbsp peanut butter

Replacements:

Coconut milk for filtered water

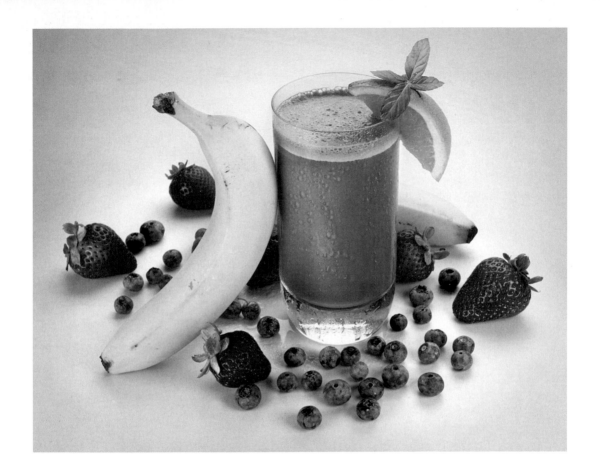

Recipe #24: Powdered Berry Joy

Tags: Beginner, Quick

Ingredients:

1 frozen banana
½ cup frozen blueberries

½ cup frozen raspberries
1 fresh peeled orange
1 scoop of flaxseed powder
1 cup filtered water

....

Recipe #25: Miessence Radical Beauty

Tags: Beginner

Ingredients:

1 frozen banana
1 cup frozen blueberries
1 cup fresh spinach
1 scoop of Miessence Berry Radical powder
1 peeled orange
1 cup filtered water

Replacements:

Use your favorite meal replacement or protein powder instead

....

Recipe #26: Multi Nutri Raw Power

Tags: Meal Replacement

Ingredients:

1 scoop Raw Warrior Rice Protein Powder
1 tsp chia seeds or powder
1 small cucumber

1 frozen avocado
1 cup frozen pineapple
1 cup fresh kale without stem
1 cup filtered water

Optional additions:

1 small chunk of ginger

Replacements:

Spinach for kale

....

Recipe #27: Almond Spice Crush

Tags: Meal Replacement, Beginner

Ingredients:

1 frozen banana
1 cup almond milk
3 tbsp Living Harvest Vanilla Chai Hemp Protein Powder
1 tbsp almond butter

....

Recipe #28: Raw Banango Spin

Tags: Hidden Green, Meal Replacement

Ingredients:

½ frozen banana
⅔ cup frozen blueberries

2 cups fresh spinach
½ cup frozen mango
1 scoop Raw Warrior Rice Protein Powder
1 tbsp hemp seeds (Hemp Hearts or other brand)
1 cup filtered water

Replacements:

Use your favorite meal replacement or protein powder instead

Recipe #29: Cacao Vanilla Shake

Tags: Beginner, Quick

Ingredients:

1 scoop raw cacao powder
1 cup almond vanilla milk
1 frozen banana
1 tbsp almond butter

Replacements:

Use your favorite unsweetened nut milk

Recipe #30: Brave Dandelion Buzz

Tags: Green Lover, Quick

Ingredients:

2 cups fresh dandelions
1 frozen banana
1 medium size apple
1 tbsp hemp seeds
1 cup filtered water

Optional additions:

A small chunk of ginger

Recipe #31: Slow Carb Super Boost

Tags: Meal Replacement, Beginner

Ingredients:

2 cups fresh spinach
½ frozen peeled avocado
1 cup almond coconut milk
2–3 ice cubes
1 tbsp almond butter
½ tsp cinnamon
1 tsp hemp seeds

Replacements:

Use your favorite unsweetened nut milk

Recipe #32: Peachy Warrior

Tags: Meal Replacement, Quick

Ingredients:

1 frozen banana
1 fresh pitted peach
1 scoop Raw Warrior Rice Protein Powder
1 cup almond milk

Optional additions:

1 tbsp flaxseed meal

Replacements:

Use any other protein powder instead

Recipe #33: Purple Oat Berry Blast

Tags: Hidden Green, Beginner, Low Fruit

Ingredients:

½ cup gluten-free rolled oats
1½ cup almond coconut milk
1 cup fresh spinach
3–4 frozen strawberries
½ cup frozen blueberries

Optional additions:

1 tbsp peanut butter or almond butter

Notes:

Soak ½ cup of gluten-free rolled oats in 1 cup almond coconut milk overnight (six to eight hours). Pour into blender and cover with ½ cup more almond coconut milk, then make smoothie.

Recipe #34: Goji Berry Almond Puree

Tags: Meal Replacement, Beginner

Ingredients:

1 cup almond milk
⅓ cup goji berries

½ to 1 cups frozen raspberries
1 scoop Dairy Free SP Complete protein powder by Standard Process
1 tbsp almond butter

Replacements:

Use any other protein powder instead

....

Recipe #35: Sweet Creamy Delight

Tags: Detox & Cleanse, Green Lover

Ingredients:

½ large frozen peeled avocado
1 cup fresh pineapple
2 cups spinach
1 handful fresh parsley
1 handful fresh mint
1 cup filtered water

....

Recipe #36: Greens All the Way

Tags: Green Lover, Quick, Low Fruit

Ingredients:

1 small frozen avocado
2 cups fresh spinach

15–20 white grapes
1 handful fresh basil
¼ cup sunflower seeds
½ lime, juiced into the blender
1 cup filtered water

Optional additions:

1 small chunk of peeled ginger

Replacements:

Mint for basil

....

Recipe #37: The Hawaiian Pink

Tags: Meal Replacement, Beginner

Ingredients:

½ cup gluten-free rolled oats
1 cup coconut milk
1 cup fresh pineapple
4 frozen strawberries
1 tbsp peanut butter

Optional additions:

1 tsp hemp seeds

Replacements:

Almond butter for peanut butter

Notes:

Soak ½ cup of gluten-free rolled oats in 1 cup coconut milk overnight (six to eight hours). Pour into blender and cover with ½ cup more coconut milk, then make smoothie.

....

Recipe #38: Chocolate Raspberry Tart

Tags: Meal Replacement, Quick, Beginner

Ingredients:

1 frozen banana
1 cup almond milk
⅓ cup dried goji berries
1 cup frozen raspberries
1 portion of Amazing Grass Amazing Meal Chocolate Infusion

Optional additions:

1 tbsp almond butter

Recipe #39: Deep Green Superfood

Tags: Hidden Green, Beginner

Ingredients:

⅔ cup frozen blueberries
2 cups of fresh spinach
1 frozen banana
1 scoop of Miessence Deep Green superfood
1 cup coconut milk
1 tbsp flaxseed powder

Recipe #40: Jerry's Double Eagle Delight

Tags: Farnoosh's Signature Gem, Beginner

Ingredients:

1 cup almond milk
3–4 frozen figs
⅔ cup frozen peeled avocado
1 cup fresh spinach
1 cup fresh or frozen pineapple

Optional additions:

A scoop of your favorite protein powder

Replacements:

Romaine lettuce for spinach

....

Recipe #41: Purple Fig Explosion

Tags: Hidden Green, Farnoosh's Signature Gem, Beginner

Ingredients:

1 frozen banana
4 frozen figs
1 cup unsweetened almond milk
1 cup fresh spinach

Optional additions:

A scoop of your favorite protein powder
1 tbsp almond butter

....

Recipe #42: Vanilla Chocolate Sunset

Tags: Beginner, Quick

Ingredients:

2 scoops Raw Cacao Powder (Navitas Naturals brand)
1 cup unsweetened, vanilla-flavored almond milk
1 frozen banana
⅓ cup dried goji berries
⅓ cup frozen raspberries

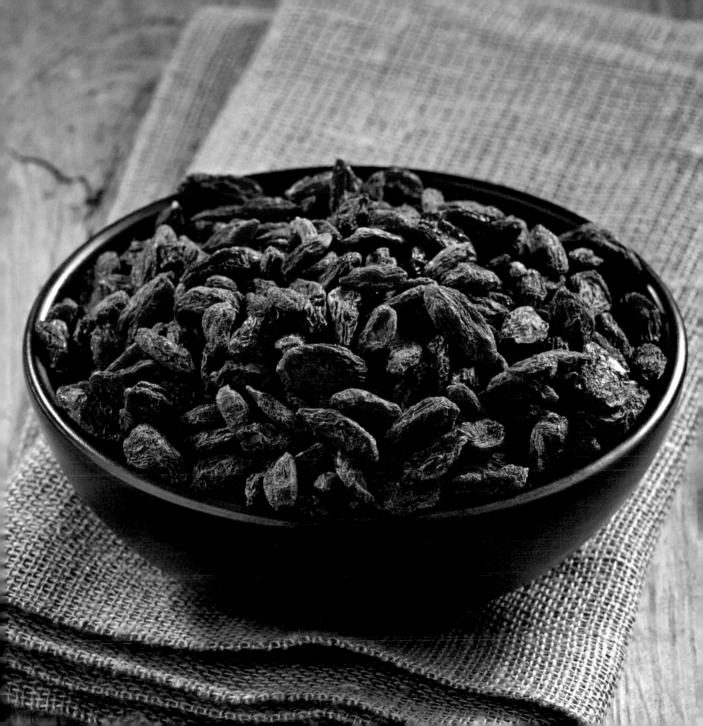

Recipe #43: Sweet Almond Oat Memento

Tags: Hidden Green, Beginner, Meal Replacement, Farnoosh's Signature Gem

Ingredients:

½ cup gluten-free rolled oats
1 cup almond milk
¼ cup water or more almond milk
½ cup frozen blueberries
3 frozen figs
1 tbsp almond butter
1 cup of fresh spinach

Optional additions:

A scoop of your favorite protein powder.

Notes:

Soak ½ cup of gluten-free rolled oats with 1 cup almond milk overnight (six to eight hours). Pour into blender and cover with ½ cup more almond milk, then make smoothie.

Recipe #44: Better than Sex Elixir

Tags: Farnoosh's Signature Gem, Beginner

Ingredients:

½ cup gluten-free rolled oats
1¼ cup almond milk

1 tbsp almond butter
1 frozen banana
4 frozen strawberries
⅓ cup frozen blueberries

Optional additions:

1 tbsp flaxseed meal

Notes:

Soak ½ cup of gluten-free rolled oats with 1 cup almond milk overnight (six to eight hours). Pour into blender and cover with ½ cup more almond milk, then make smoothie.

....

Recipe #45: The Unbelievable Fig Rapture

Tags: Quick, Meal Replacement

Ingredients:

1 frozen peeled avocado
⅓ cup fresh white grapes
4 frozen figs
3–4 fresh kale leaves without stalk
1 cup almond milk
1 tbsp almond butter

Replacements:

Spinach for kale

Recipe #46: Carrot Mango Sensation

Tags: Quick, Green Lover, Detox & Cleanse

Ingredients:

1 medium carrot
1 cup frozen mango
A small handful of parsley
6–7 leaves of romaine lettuce
1 scoop of Miessence Deep Green superfood

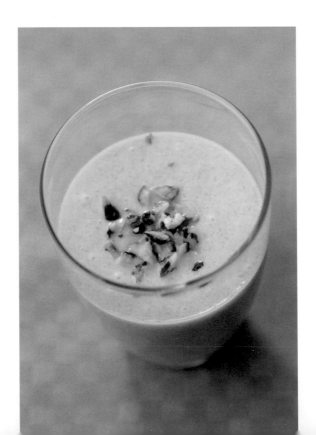

Recipe #47: The Incredibly Creamy Avocado Banana Babe

Tags: Beginner, Quick, Low Fruit

Ingredients:

1 cup fresh spinach
1 small frozen avocado
½ frozen banana
¼ cup frozen raspberries
1–1½ cup almond milk
1 tbsp flaxseed powder

Recipe #48: The Great Fig Goddess

Tags: Hidden Green, Beginner, Meal Replacement, Farnoosh's Signature Gem

Ingredients:

1–1½ cup almond milk
1 frozen banana
1 tbsp almond butter
¼ cup frozen blueberries
1 cup fresh spinach
4 frozen figs

Optional additions:

A scoop of your favorite protein powder or hemp seed powder

Recipe #49: Citrus Pear Sensation

Tags: Detox & Cleanse, Green Lover, Farnoosh's Signature Gem, Low Fruit

Ingredients:

½ frozen peeled avocado
1 green pear
1 cup fresh spinach
1 handful of fresh parsley
½ lemon, juice squeezed into the blender
1 cup filtered water

Recipe #50: The Rolled Oat Peach Energizer

Tags: Beginner

Ingredients:

½ cup gluten-free rolled oats
1–1½ cup almond milk
1 cup frozen peach chunks
1 frozen banana
1 tbsp almond butter

Optional additions:

A scoop of your favorite protein powder or hemp seed powder

Notes:

Soak ½ cup of gluten-free rolled oats with 1 cup almond coconut milk overnight (six to eight hours). Pour into blender and cover with ½ cup more almond coconut milk then add frozen fruit on top. Blend until smooth and ready.

....

Recipe #51: Peachy-Nana Pudding

Tags: Quick, Detox & Cleanse

Ingredients:

1 frozen banana
1 cup frozen peach
1½ cups fresh Swiss chard, without stalk
1 cup filtered water

Optional additions:

A scoop of your favorite protein powder or hemp seed powder
or 1 tbsp almond butter

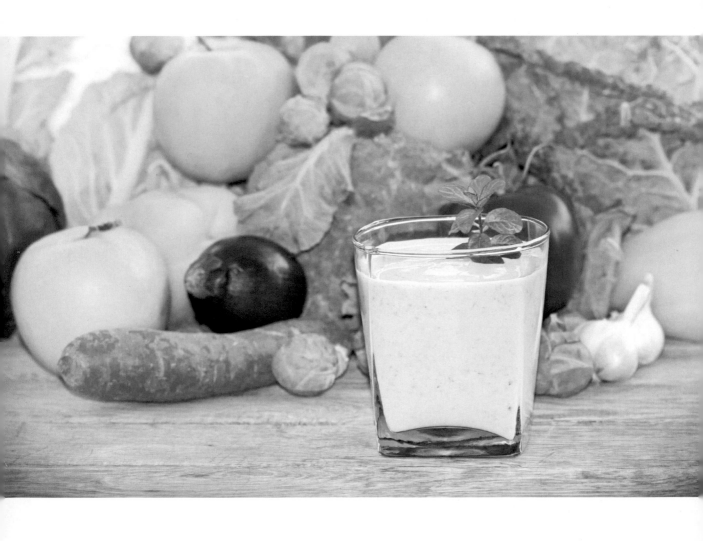

Recipe #52: The Purple Fig Swirl

Tags: Hidden Green, Meal Replacement

Ingredients:

½ cup gluten-free rolled oats
1 frozen banana
4 frozen figs
½ cup frozen blueberries
1½ cups fresh spinach and Swiss chard mix.
1 cup almond milk
1 tbsp almond butter

Optional additions:

A scoop of your favorite protein powder or hemp seed powder

Notes:

Soak ½ cup of gluten-free rolled oats with 1 cup almond coconut milk overnight (six to eight hours). Pour into blender and cover with ½ cup more almond coconut milk, then make smoothie.

Recipe #53: Chard to the Rescue

Tags: Detox & Cleanse, Green Lover, Quick

Ingredients:

3 frozen figs
½ fresh or frozen mango

½ cup frozen peach
1½ cup fresh spinach and Swiss chard
1 handful of parsley
1 cup filtered water

Recipe #54: Healthy Heart Breakfast

Tags: Green Lover, Quick

1½ cup kale, no stem
1 handful of fresh mint
1 frozen banana
½ large pear
1 tbsp hemp seeds
1 cup filtered water

Optional additions:

A chunk of ginger

Recipe #55: The Hawaiian Paradiso

Tags: Meal Replacement, Quick

½ cup frozen raspberries
1 frozen peeled avocado
1½ cup fresh spinach
2 tbsp coconut shreds
1 cup coconut milk

1 tbsp almond butter

Optional additions:

A scoop of your favorite protein powder

. . . .

Recipe #56: Coco-Kiwi Island Bliss

Tags: Meal Replacement, Beginner, Low Fruit

1 frozen peeled avocado
1½ cup fresh spinach
2 tbsp coconut shreds
1 tbsp hemp seeds
1 cup coconut almond milk
1½ frozen peeled kiwi

Optional additions:

A scoop of your favorite protein powder

Replacements:

Frozen banana instead of avocado, or do half and half of each

Recipe #57: Limy Minty Charm

Tags: Detox & Cleanse, Farnoosh's Signature Gem, Green Lover

1 orange, peeled
½ fresh lime, juice squeezed into the blender
1 cup frozen pineapple

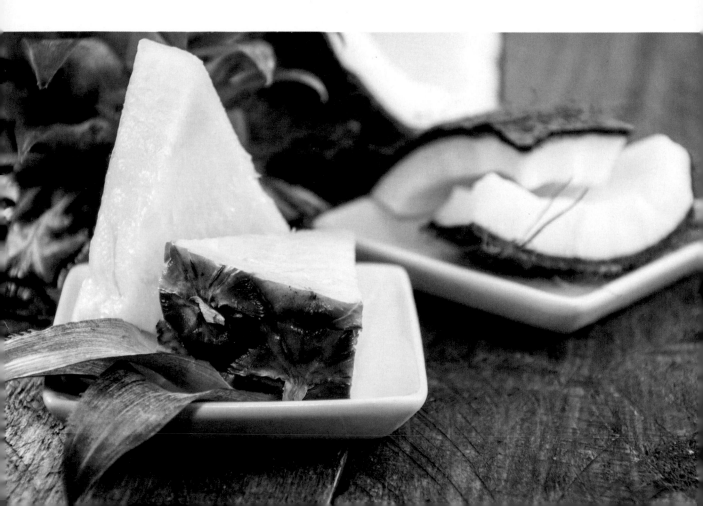

1 handful parsley
1½ cups fresh spinach
1 small handful fresh mint

Optional additions:

1 small chunk of ginger

Recipe #58: Yummy Date with Love

Tags: Beginner, Low Fruit

1½ cups almond coconut milk
1 small frozen avocado, peeled
1 large handful of fresh spinach
2 pitted dates
1 tbsp flaxseed powder

Optional additions:

A scoop of your favorite protein powder

Recipe #59: Spinach Meets Cinnamon

Tags: Quick, Green Lover

1¼ cups almond coconut milk
1–2 stalks of celery
1 handful of spinach

2 pitted dates
1 frozen banana
½ tsp cinnamon

Optional additions:

A scoop of your favorite protein powder

....

Recipe #60: A Smooth Coconut Treat

Tags: Quick, Green Lover

1¼ cups almond coconut milk
1 handful of spinach
2 pitted dates
1–2 celery stalks
1 frozen avocado
½ fresh apple
1 tbsp flaxseed powder

....

Recipe #61: Before Sunrise Glee

Tags: Beginner, Low Fruit

1¼ cups almond milk
½ cup of soaked oats
1 fresh de-cored apple
¼ tsp cinnamon

Optional additions:

1 frozen avocado

Notes:

Soak the oats in ½ cup of almond milk overnight. Then add the rest of almond milk, the apple and cinnamon, and the frozen avocado as optional on top and blend until smooth and ready.

....

Recipe #62: Cabba-Berry Thrill

Tags: Hidden Green, Low Fruit, Beginner

1 cup coconut milk
1½ cups fresh white cabbage
½ fresh avocado
½ cup frozen blueberries
¼ tsp cinnamon

Optional additions:

1 tbsp almond butter

Replacements:

Use strawberries in place of blueberries.

Notes:

Add the coconut milk and the cabbage to the blender first, then avocado, nut butter, and blueberries on top. Blend until smooth and ready.

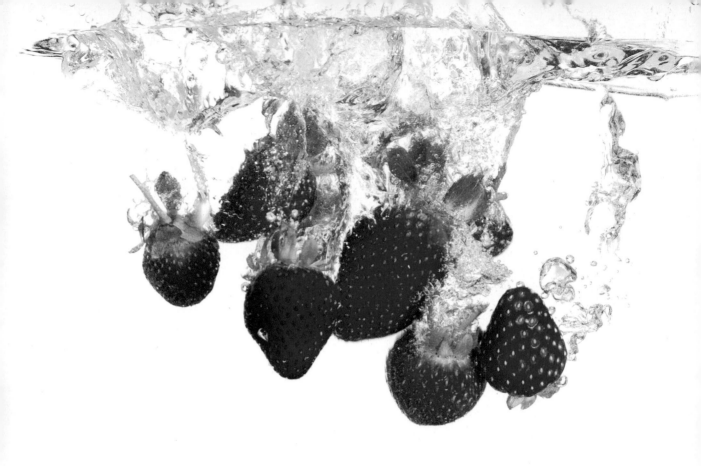

Recipe #63: Acai-Mango Healer

Tags: Beginner

1 cup almond-coconut milk
½-⅔ cup gluten-free rolled oats, soaked
½ cup frozen mangos

178

½ cup or 3 frozen strawberries
1 tbsp acai powder
¼ cup filtered water

Notes:

Soak ½ cup of gluten-free rolled oats with 1 cup almond coconut milk overnight (six to eight hours). Pour into blender and cover with ½ cup more almond coconut milk, then make smoothie.

Recipe #64: Vanilla Cabbage Concoction

Tags: Hidden Green, Beginner

1¼ cups almond milk
1 ½ cup shredded or cup fresh cabbage
1 large frozen banana
1 tbsp hemp seeds
1 tbsp almond butter

Optional additions:

⅛ teaspoon vanilla extract

Recipe #65: Pineapple Spinach Blast

Tags: Beginner, Quick

1¼ cups coconut milk

1 frozen large banana
1 cup frozen pineapple
2 cups baby spinach
2 tbsp flaxseed powder

Optional additions:

¼ tsp vanilla extract

Recipe #66: Super Green Glow

Tags: Detox & Cleanse, Farnoosh's Signature Gem, Quick

1½ cups filtered water
1 small frozen banana
½ fresh apple, de-cored
½ fresh pear
1 cup baby spinach
1 cup romaine lettuce
1 lemon, juice squeezed into blender

Optional additions:

1 stalk of celery
¼ cup cilantro or parsley

Replacements:

All spinach for all lettuce

Recipe #67: Oh My God Delicious

Tags: Beginner, Quick

1 cup coconut milk
¼ cup shredded coconut
1 celery stalk
1 handful fresh parsley
½ fresh pear
1 frozen banana

Recipe #68: Spicy Sweet Potato Shake

Tags: Beginner, Low Fruit

1¼ cups almond milk
⅔-1 cup cooked mashed chilled sweet potato
¼ tsp turmeric
¾ tsp cinnamon
2 ice cubes
1 tbsp almond butter

Replacements:

Use cooked mashed pumpkin instead of sweet potato

Notes:

Bake sweet potato in the oven, remove peel, chill in the fridge for two hours or more, then add to blender to make the recipe.

Recipe #69: Hemp Me Out

Tags: Meal Replacement, Beginner, Quick

1 cup coconut milk
2 tbsp Living Harvest Hemp Protein Original Flavor
1 frozen banana
2 tbsp raw cacao powder
4 ice cubes

Replacements:

Use your own favorite protein powder. Choose a neutral flavor.

Recipe #70: Green Clue to Life

Tags: Green Lover, Farnoosh's Signature Gem, Detox & Cleanse

1½ cups filtered water
2 stalks of celery
1 handful fresh mint
1 handful fresh parsley
1 lemon, juice squeezed into blender
1 red apple, de-cored
½ pear
1 frozen banana

Replacements:

Use your own favorite protein powder. Use a neutral flavor.

Recipe #71: High Vitamin Infusion

Tags: Green Lover, Quick

1½ cups filtered water
1½ cups chopped collard greens
1 Granny Smith Apple
½ frozen banana
½ fresh pear
½ fresh squeezed lemon
1 handful fresh mint
1 tbsp flaxseed powder
½ tbsp chia powder

Recipe #72: An Unlikely Combination

Tags: Green Lover, Meal Replacement

1½ cups of almond coconut milk
½ cup gluten-free rolled oats
4–5 stems of dandelions
4–5 stems of parsley
A small handful of spinach
2 pitted dates
3 frozen strawberries
1 frozen banana

Optional additions:

1 tbsp chia seeds

Recipe #73: Drink Your Salad

Tags: Detox & Cleanse, Green Lover, Farnoosh's Signature Gem, Low Fruit

1 cup filtered water
6 ice cubes
½ fresh avocado
1 medium tomato, Roma or Heirloom
1–2 cloves of garlic
1 small handful mint
2 broccoli florets
1 handful fresh parsley
½ green bell pepper, no seeds
½ lime, juice squeezed into blender

Optional additions:

A pinch of kosher salt

Replacements:

Celery for broccoli

Recipe #74: Ultimate Salad Medley

Tags: Detox & Cleanse, Meal Replacement, Green Lover, Low Fruit

1 cup filtered water
6 ice cubes
½ fresh avocado

1 medium tomato, Roma or Heirloom
1–2 cloves of garlic
½ Italian cucumber
4 stalks of dandelion
1 handful fresh baby kale
4 broccoli florets, no stem
½ green bell pepper, no seeds
1 lemon, juice squeezed into blender

Optional additions:

1 tbsp raw sesame seeds
A dash of extra virgin olive oil

Recipe #75: Almond Coconut Ecstasy

Tags: Quick, Beginner, Meal Replacement

1 cup almond coconut milk
1 frozen or fresh banana
1 frozen pitted peach
2 pitted dates
1 handful fresh spinach
1 scoop of Raw Power Raw Warrior Brown Rice Protein Powder

Optional additions:

Chia powder or flaxseed powder

Notes:

Soak ½ cup of gluten-free rolled oats with 1 cup almond milk overnight (six to eight hours). Pour into blender and cover with ½ cup more almond milk, then make smoothie.

....

Recipe #76: Spicy Green Salad

Tags: Green Lover, Detox & Cleanse, Low Fruit

½ cup filtered water
5–6 ice cubes
1 medium tomato, Roma or Heirloom
1 handful fresh parsley
1 handful fresh baby kale
½ habanero pepper without seeds
½ Italian cucumber
1 cup of fresh white cabbage
1 lemon juice squeezed into blender

Optional additions:

Dash of cayenne pepper
1–2 tbsp sunflower seeds

Replacements:

Use any of your favorite greens in place of baby kale and parsley

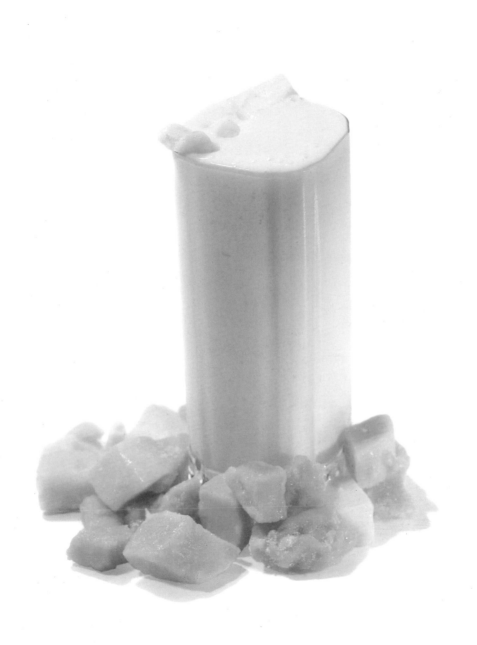

Recipe #77: Dandelion Mango Party

Tags: Hidden Green, Meal Replacement

1 cup almond milk
¼ to ½ cup filtered water
4–5 leaves of dandelions
½ cup gluten-free rolled oats
½ cup frozen mango
1 frozen banana
1 tbsp acai powder

Replacements:

Any favorite greens for dandelions

Notes:

Soak ½ cup of gluten-free rolled oats with 1 cup almond coconut milk overnight (six to eight hours). Pour into blender and cover with ½ cup more almond coconut milk, then make smoothie.

Recipe #78: Saffron Pistachio Persian Delight

Tags: Farnoosh's Signature Gem, Low Fruit, Hidden Green

1/16 tsp or a pinch of saffron
2 pitted dates
1 handful fresh spinach
¼ cup pistachios without shells

½ tsp vanilla extract
1 cup almond milk
½ cup cooked chilled jasmine rice
4 cubes of ice

Replacements:

Use coconut milk or coconut almond milk.

Notes:

Soak saffron in ⅛ cup hot water for two hours. Cook jasmine rice using your rice cooker or the stove. Measure and chill ½ cup cooked rice. Pour pistachios into the blender first, run the blender for 30 seconds to powderize the nuts. Add rice, almond milk, and the other ingredients and blend until smooth and ready.

....

Recipe #79: Rocket in My Smoothie

Tags: Meal Replacement, Hidden Green

1 cup almond milk
1 handful of arugula (rocket)
½-1 frozen banana
½ frozen peach, pitted
½ fresh apple
1 tbsp almond butter
1 healthy dash of cinnamon

Recipe #80: Citrus Fennel Pudding

Tags: Detox & Cleanse, Farnoosh's Signature Gem, Green Lover

1½ cups filtered water
3–4 ice cubes
½ frozen avocado
1 green apple
½ pear
1 handful baby kale, no stem
1 celery stalk
¼ fennel bulb and stalk
½ lemon, juice squeezed into blender

Optional additions:

1 tbsp sesame seeds

Replacements:

Spinach or Swiss chard for kale

Recipe #81: Persia Meets Japan

Tags: Farnoosh's Signature Gem, Beginner

1¼ cups almond milk
½ cup of soaked oats
⅛ cup pistachios
⅛ cup goji berries

½ tsp Matcha tea powder
1 frozen banana
3 frozen strawberries

Optional additions:

⅛ to ¼ tsp of vanilla extract

Notes:

Soak ½ cup of gluten-free rolled oats with 1 cup almond coconut milk overnight (six to eight hours). Pour into blender and cover with ½ cup more almond coconut milk, then make smoothie.

....

Recipe #82: Matcha Doing

Tags: Meal Replacement, Farnoosh's Signature Gem

1 cup almond milk
½ cup of soaked oats
½ tsp Matcha tea powder
2 pitted dates
1 frozen banana
⅛ cup pistachios
1 handful of spinach
⅛ cup frozen raspberries
¼ cup filtered water

Replacements:

Use any brand of almond milk, with or without vanilla flavor

Notes:

Soak ½ cup of oats in 1 cup of almond milk overnight. Then add the pistachios, Matcha tea, and frozen fruit last. Blend until smooth and ready.

....

Recipe #83: Uber Hydrating Cooler

Tags: Detox & Cleanse, Green Lover

1–1½ cups filtered water
6 ice cubes
1 handful baby kale, no stem
4–5 leaves basil, no stem
4–5 leaves dandelion
⅛ of a funnel bulb
½ apple
½ pear
½ lemon, juice squeezed into blender
A small chunk of peeled fresh ginger

Replacements:

Use any desired combination of the greens

....

Recipe #84: Fruitless Fantasy

Tags: Detox & Cleanse, Green Lover, Low Fruit

1 cup filtered water
1 medium carrot, without the carrot top

2 small cucumbers
1 large tomato or 2 Roma tomatoes
2 cups broccoli florets
1–2 cloves garlic, peeled
1 frozen avocado
½ lime, juice squeezed into blender

Optional additions:

½ habanero or jalapeno pepper, without seeds
⅛ cup sunflower seeds

Recipe #85: Carrot Banana Blend

Tags: Hidden Green, Detox & Cleanse

1 medium carrot
½ frozen banana
1–2 celery stalk
1 medium apple, de-cored
1 handful (4–5) carrot tops
1½ cups filtered water
½ juice of lime squeezed into blender

Replacements:

Parsley for carrot tops

Recipe #86: Ocean Blue Almond Fusion

Tags: Farnoosh's Signature Gem, Meal Replacement

1 tsp spirulina
1 frozen banana
1 cup frozen pineapple chunks
1¼ cups almond milk
1 tbsp almond butter
1 tbsp hemp seeds

Recipe #87: Feed Me Darling

Tags: Hidden Green, Farnoosh's Signature Gem

1 cup almond milk
½ cup oats soaked
1 small frozen banana
½ cup frozen pineapple chunks
3 fresh or frozen strawberries
4 large romaine lettuce leaves
1 tsp spirulina

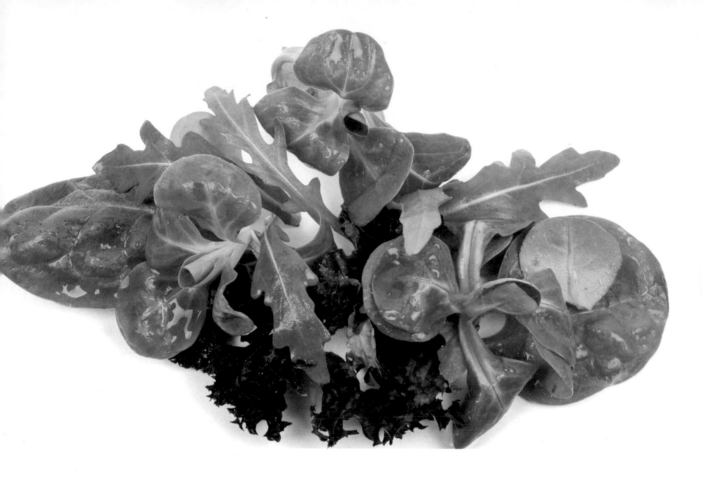

Recipe #88: Red Pomo-Mango Elation

Tags: Beginner, Quick

1 cup almond milk
1 handful fresh spinach
½ cup fresh or frozen pomegranate seeds

½ cup frozen mango
½ fresh apple
1 tbsp flaxseed powder

....

Recipe #89: Vibrant Green Joy

Tags: Low Fruit, Green Lover, Detox & Cleanse

1 cup filtered water
1 small handful cilantro
1 frozen avocado
2–3 carrot tops
1–2 leaves of romaine lettuce
3 frozen or fresh strawberries
½ cup fresh pomegranate seeds
½ lemon, juice squeezed into blender

Optional additions:

A pinch of sea salt

Replacements:

Parsley for cilantro
Swiss chard or spinach for carrot tops

Recipe #90: Blue Green Ocean

Tags: Farnoosh's Signature Gem, Meal Replacement

1½ cups almond milk
½ cup gluten-free oats
2 pitted dates
¼ cup frozen pomegranate seeds
1 frozen banana
2 frozen strawberries
1 tsp spirulina

Replacements:

Use coconut milk in place of almond milk.

Recipe #91: Orange Zesty Elixir

Tags: Beginner, Farnoosh's Signature Gem, Detox & Cleanse

1 cup filtered water
1 frozen banana
1 peeled orange
½ apple
1 large handful spinach

Optional additions:

1 small chunk of ginger, peeled

Recipe #92: Happiness Extract

Tags: Meal Replacement, Farnoosh's Signature Gem

1 cup almond milk
1–2 tsp acai powder
½ cup frozen mangos
½ fresh pear
2 frozen strawberries
½ cup soaked gluten-free oats
1 tbsp almond butter

Recipe #93: Cool Me Down Orange Cukes

Tags: Detox & Cleanse, Quick

¼ cup water
3–4 ice cubes
1 orange peeled
½ fresh pear
1 small cucumber or ⅓ of a large Italian cucumber

Optional additions:

½ lime, juice squeezed into the blender
¼ cup fresh cranberries

Recipe #94: Guilt-Free Chocolate Raspberry Joy

Tags: Beginner, Quick

1½ cups almond milk
1 frozen banana
3–4 frozen strawberries
¼ cup frozen raspberries
2 pitted dates
1 tbsp raw cacao powder

Optional additions:

A pinch of cinnamon

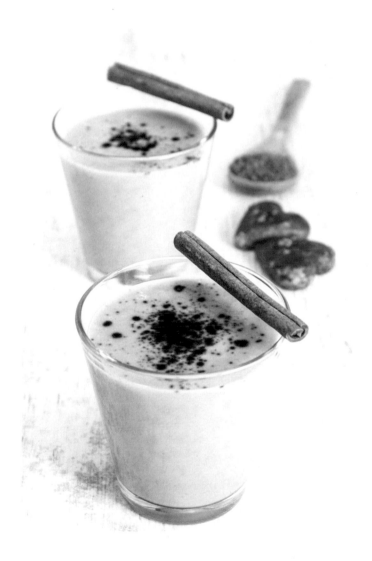

Recipe #95: Cacao Berry Distraction

Tags: Quick, Low Fruit

1 cup almond milk
5 medium frozen strawberries
½ frozen avocado
2 tbsp raw cacao powder
A dash of cinnamon
2 scoops of Standard Process Protein Powder

Replacements:

Use your own favorite protein powder

Recipe #96: Crystal Green Lagoon

Tags: Detox & Cleanse, Green Lover, Quick

1 cup filtered water
1 frozen banana
1 frozen kiwi, peeled
½ fresh pear
4–5 leaves kale, no stalk
½ lemon, juice squeezed into blender

Optional additions:

1 dash cinnamon

Recipe #97: Out of This World

Tags: Green Lover, Detox & Cleanse, Farnoosh's Signature Gem

1 cup filtered water
½ frozen or fresh peeled mango
⅛ fennel bulb
1–1½ stalks celery
2 large leaves of green Swiss chard
2 pitted dates
1 dash cinnamon

Recipe #98: Pink Sweet Babe

Tags: Beginner, Quick

1 persimmon, unpeeled
1½ frozen bananas
¼ cup cranberries
2 pitted dates
1½ cups filtered water

Optional additions:

2 dashes cinnamon

Recipe #99: Pear with Me

Tags: Detox & Cleanse, Farnoosh's Signature Gem, Beginner

1 cup filtered water
2 large leaves of green Swiss chard
1 frozen kiwi
½ fresh pear
1 peeled orange
½ frozen banana

Recipe #100: For the Love of Avocado

Tags: Beginner, Low Fruit, Quick

1 cup filtered water
2 large leaves of green Swiss chard
½ lime juice squeezed into the blender
½ fresh pear
1 small frozen avocado
1 tbsp flaxseed powder

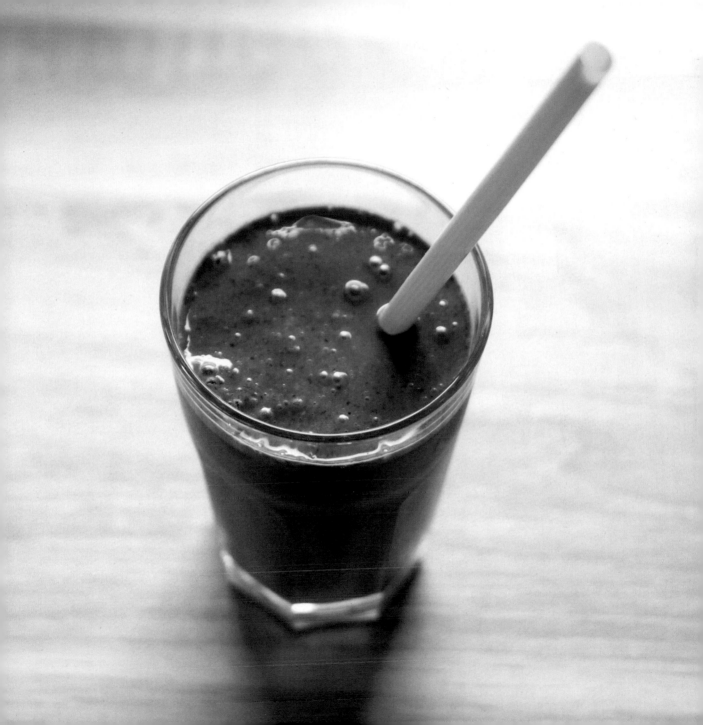

Recipe #101: So Green So Good

Tags: Detox & Cleanse, Green Lover, Hidden Green, Quick

1 cup filtered water
½ cup frozen blueberries
½ fresh mango
½ fresh pear
1 frozen banana
1 handful fresh spinach
1 handful fresh parsley

Recipe #102: Pom Pom Delight

Tags: Detox & Cleanse, Beginner, Farnoosh's Signature Gem

1½ cups filtered water
5 ice cubes
1½ fresh banana
¼ cup frozen pomegranate seeds
1 orange, peeled
2 pitted dates
3–4 leaves Swiss chard

Recipe #103: Matcha Rising Sun

Tags: Farnoosh's Signature Gem

1 cup brewed chilled Matcha tea
4–5 ice cubes
1 small fresh avocado
1 orange, peeled
½ large apple
A large handful romaine lettuce

Optional additions:

A dash or two of cinnamon

Recipe #104: The Green Dragon

Tags: Green Lover, Detox & Cleanse

1 handful fresh parsley
3–4 Swiss chard leaves
1 frozen mango
⅔ cup frozen blueberries
½ fresh pear
½ lemon, juice squeezed into the blender

Recipe #105: Blue Goji Mamma

Tags: Low Fruit, Quick

1½ cups almond milk
1 handful fresh spinach
½ frozen avocado
⅓ cup frozen raspberries
⅓ cup frozen goji berries
½ tsp spirulina

Recipe #106: Polka Dot Berry Dance

Tags: Low Fruit, Hidden Green

1½ cup almond milk
1 handful fresh spinach
⅓ cup frozen blueberries
⅓ cup frozen blackberries
1 tbsp chia seeds or powder

Optional additions:

A scoop of your own favorite protein powder

Notes:

Soak ½ cup of gluten-free rolled oats in 1 cup almond milk overnight (six to eight hours). Pour into blender and cover with ½ cup more almond milk, then make smoothie.

Recipe #107: Passion Hydrating Potion

Tags: Beginner, Quick, Detox & Cleanse

½-⅔ cup frozen pineapple
¼ cup frozen blueberries
¼ cup frozen cranberries
1 small cucumber
1 cup filtered water
3–4 ice cubes

Recipe #108: The Peaceful Warrior

Tags: Beginner, Quick, Detox & Cleanse, Farnoosh's Signature Gem

1–2 small cucumbers
1 cup frozen pineapple chunks
4–5 Romaine lettuce leaves
¼ cup frozen pomegranate seeds
1 cup filtered water

Optional additions:

½ lemon, juice squeezed into the blender

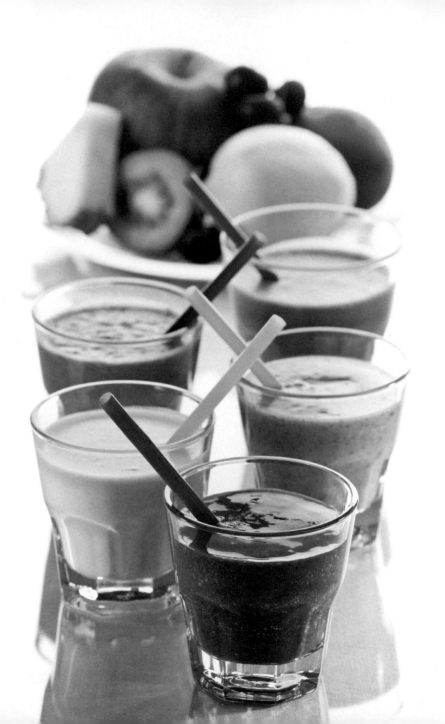

A Smoothie Beauty Detox & Cleanse Plan

He that takes medicine and neglects diet wastes the skill of the physician.
~Chinese Proverb

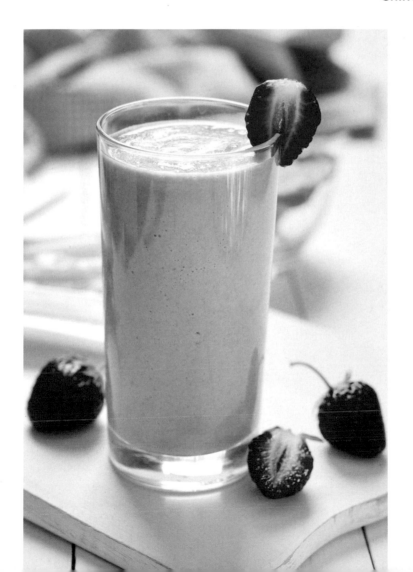

Smoothies are healthy, delicious, full of nutrients, and fun to make. You know that by now, but what you may not know is that they are the perfect beauty drink. They bring a glow to your skin and a new shine to your hair. They return the spark back to once-tired eyes and wipe out fatigue, which adversely affects your natural beauty. Say it with me: Smoothies are my beauty food, baby!

To help you go deeper in this beauty path with smoothies, I created an easy-to-follow Detox & Cleanse program for you. I have already done the program myself, and I return to it whenever I need a nice reboot and rejuvenation to my system. For me, that time is usually after a lot of travel and flying around in airplanes. If you are away from home and especially from your kitchen a lot, then use a weekend at home as a great time to do this. The results can last for weeks, and you will have renewed motivation for taking your smoothie habit to a higher level. Let's Detox & Cleanse together, shall we?

Detox & Cleanse Smoothie Plans

Leave your drugs in the chemist's pot if you can heal the patient with food.
~Hippocrates

I am a huge fan of natural cleanses. In *The Healthy Juicer's Bible*, I talk about juice fasting in great detail as a great way to achieve extreme detox and cleanse results, and here we talk about using healthy smoothies to achieve similar results. I do not recommend expensive medication, surgery, colonic therapy, or anything that is going to take you outside your kitchen and into a medicine cabinet or doctor's chair. Your body can heal itself. Help it. Nudge it in the right direction with nature's superfoods. The gentle approach with smoothies is effective, budget-friendly, natural, and it works.

First, let's define the term "Detox & Cleanse." This refers to the act of removing accumulated waste and toxins from your body. Your body itself is a beautiful machine, and as long as you have a functioning kidney, liver, and colon, your body is removing waste and keeping you nice and clean on the inside, but when you are putting a lot of toxins in your body with a poor diet, these functions may slow down. Healthy smoothies help reverse the process and help your body return to its natural detoxification in a gentle way.

One way to think of Detox & Cleanse is to reduce or completely eliminate the bad foods that you consume, such as refined sugars, alcohol, caffeine, and chemicals such as MSG, pesticides, food colorings, tobacco, and unnecessary medications. If you have been eating an unhealthy diet for a long time, and then go on a smoothie, raw food, or juice detox, your body may initially show detox symptoms such as skin breakouts, gas, bloating, head fogginess, grumpiness, headaches, joint ache, constipation, and diarrhea. You may also use the bathroom a lot more than usual, which can be a great relief but might need some planning ahead with your daily schedules.

So How Does a Detox & Cleanse with Smoothies Work?

With healthy and especially super green smoothies, you are pumping tons of nutrients and fiber into your body in a form that is readily digestible. The calories fill you up and take care of hunger, while the fiber helps flush out the waste. The nutrients help your skin, and the overall effect allows your body and your organs to return to their natural harmony.

Fruits are water-rich and full of nutrients and vitamins, especially vitamin C. They are also incredibly easy for your body to digest—they quickly pass through your system, especially in the blended puréed form. Fruits help your digestive system to work super efficiently because they put little to no strain on it. Fruit is brilliant for cleansing by itself. And greens are Mother Nature's jewel. They are rich in chlorophyll, a substance in plants that purifies the blood and cleanses the body.

Both fruits and vegetables give you plenty of good fiber. When you combine these two, you are creating a superfood, natural detox drink that cannot begin to compare with anything in a pill or on a shelf. Your smoothie is your superfood, as I've already said a few times. It is a food that has none of the "bad stuff" for your body, and it is filled to the brim with the "good stuff." You are shifting the inside scales of your body in the right direction with each green healthy smoothie.

Should you do a Detox & Cleanse? I would say that you can only gain benefits from it. If you want a complete overhaul of your system, if you want to reboot and restart fresh with your body and your overall nutrition, and if you have been neglecting self-care and proper nutrition for six months or longer, then a Detox & Cleanse can be extremely beneficial as well as motivating to get you started on your smoothie journey. Please check with your doctor before going on this regimen, especially if you have any special conditions, such as diabetes or pregnancy.

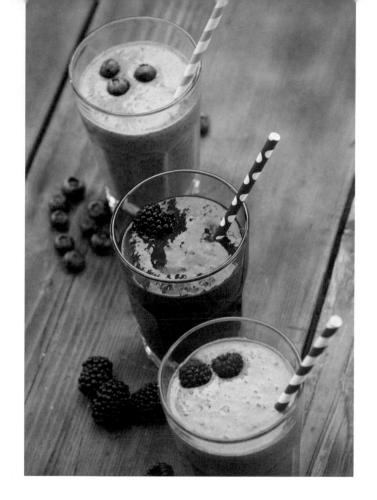

What to Eat and Drink During a Smoothie Detox & Cleanse Regimen?

During the Detox & Cleanse regimen, you want to consume only green smoothies with natural fruits and vegetables. Don't worry; you will get plenty of calories from your smoothies and won't go hungry. The Detox & Cleanse obstacles are 99 percent mental, 1 percent physical. All you have to do is get your brain on board. The rest is easy.

Here is what you can consume on your short Detox & Cleanse regimen:

1. Water
2. Healthy smoothie (preferably green): Containing only organic fresh fruits, vegetables, and greens.
3. Optional: Loose leaf tea or black coffee

You can use frozen fruit if you have frozen it yourself or know that there are no additional preservatives in the fruit packages. If possible during your detox, opt to get everything as organic.

A note on the caffeine debate: I have to say that it is a personal choice. I do not subscribe to the theory that a moderate amount of caffeine from high-quality tea and coffee is "bad" for you. In fact, high-quality loose leaf organic teas, such as green teas, are excellent source of antioxidants and help with flushing out your systems and keeping you warm during a detox. I am no longer a coffee drinker; I prefer tea and drink plenty of it. If you are in love with your cuppa joe, just beware

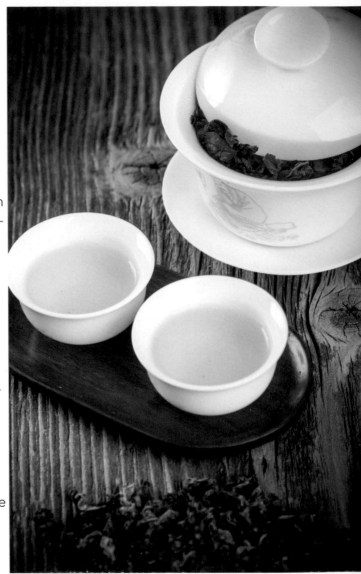

that giving up the caffeine will add withdrawal challenges to your Detox & Cleanse. But if you are a real trooper, then go sans caffeine by all means.

You can drink as much smoothie as you like during your Detox & Cleanse. Remember, there is no such thing as going hungry during the detox. Do not deprive yourself. I drink between 160 to 200 ounces of healthy smoothie during a detox, sometimes more. Of course, a good portion of that is filtered water, which is used for smoothie base, as well as the water-rich fruits and vegetables. But I do not limit myself at all. In fact, I truly enjoy drinking my green smoothie during this time. The greener you make your smoothies, the better. I recommend adding greens to more than half of your smoothies and ideally to *all* of your smoothies during the Detox & Cleanse.

What to Avoid During a Detox Regimen

These are ingredients that you may add to your smoothies at other times, but if you are doing a Detox & Cleanse, do not use them. The main reason behind it is simple: Adding any of these ingredients slows down the digestive process. Even if they can be good for your body, the goal is to lessen the efforts on the digestive system so it can get rid of accumulated waste and not work hard on new foods coming into the body.

So avoid the following during the Detox & Cleanse period:

1. Powdered superfoods and protein powders
2. Oils, such as coconut oil or flaxseed oil
3. Fats such as coconut, nuts, and seeds
4. Nut milks or other liquids for base

Suggested Detox & Cleanse Regimens

You can do a three-day, five-day, seven-day or ten-day smoothie Detox & Cleanse. I would recommend you start with a three-day and see how you feel. I also do not recommend you go longer than ten days without any solid food. Of course, after the cleanse, you will continue drinking your green smoothies in addition to other foods. The idea is to come out of your Detox & Cleanse with a much better sense of how you nourish your body.

What I love about Detox & Cleanse regimens is the simplicity of it. Diets and nutritional programs can get so complicated. Simplicity can be such a breath of fresh air. You just drink your favorite healthy (green!) smoothie, rotate your greens, mix it up as you like. The only rule is to stick to *only* fruits and veggies in your smoothie, drink plenty of water and make your own decisions on moderate amounts of caffeine.

A few quick tips for a successful Detox & Cleanse:

1. Schedule it for when you have some time to yourself and a low-key social calendar.
2. Do this when you are close to home and with plenty of access to your kitchen.
3. Do this in a warmer season the first time. Spring or fall is perfect. Avoid winter.
4. Plan your recipes in advance and do your shopping at the beginning of the week.
5. Prepare your kitchen and your refrigerator by removing all tempting foods and if possible, do not cook for others during this time or spend time in restaurants or other social circles around food.
6. Keep a smoothie journal to note how you feel and any detox symptoms (good or bad) that you may experience. Review only after the regimen is finished.
7. Set aside a non-food reward to give yourself upon completion of your Detox & Cleanse.

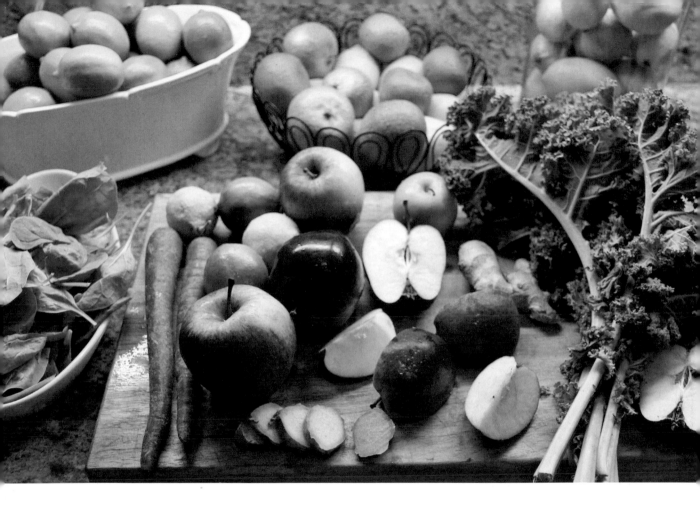

What to Expect From Your Detox & Cleanse?

There is no hard and fast rule on how to do something. These are only guidelines and best practices. As I write this section for you, I'm in the middle of another three-day Detox & Cleanse, and I've had a fresh reminder on just how challenging day one of every detox can be. Same as with juice fasting, somewhere around midday on day one of your

Detox & Cleanse with smoothies, your body will go through moodiness, grumpiness, and cravings for solid food. You'll come up with every reason under the sun to break out of it. Resist the temptation!

Stay the course by making sure you have had plenty of smoothie to keep you full. Drink some water. Get out of the kitchen. Go read a book, take a hot bath, distract yourself, and go to bed early. Day two is always much better, and you'll have plenty of energy to carry you through the day. By day three, you'll begin to feel really good and see some good results.

Now, if you are absolutely miserable, then go as long as you think you can and consider a change of plans. Remember, you are the boss. You have to make the call as to whether it's too stressful for you to continue. Are you at a point that you just can't stand the thought of another smoothie? Then call it a short cleanse and celebrate with a raw salad without dressing or a piece of fruit such as an apple, a banana, or some raw nuts. Even then, you are basically consuming the same food—raw fruits, raw vegetables—in unblended form. If possible, wait until the following day to have cooked foods. Always feel free to make the right modifications for you without feeling guilty. A Detox & Cleanse is about feeling good and learning about your body, your tolerances, your emotions, and your digestive system. If the first one or two tries don't go as planned, just do it again in the near future. You're still a winner!

Now listen, if you stick with it, here are the top eight Detox & Cleanse benefits from a long list that you get to enjoy:

1. Amazing surge of energy after the first 24–36 hours.
2. Lots of elimination of waste and a feeling of internal cleansing.

3. Loss of bloating, water weight, puffiness, fatigue, and body aches.
4. Extreme mental clarity and focus.
5. Deep, sound, restful sleep.
6. Skin glow from purification of body cells and organs.
7. A feeling of becoming grounded and balanced.
8. An overflow of love and celebration for your body and your being.

During the time that you do your Detox & Cleanse, it would be ideal to schedule some other activities that can enhance the experience and complement the internal work you are doing. These are some of those activities:

- Hot bath with Epsom salt or essential oils.
- Meditation once or twice a day, upon beginning your day, another upon closing it out.
- A massage or any other type of bodywork.
- Gentle exercise, such as walking or swimming or gentle yoga.
- Quiet time to read, reflect, and journal about the experience.
- A break from social media, TV, the news, and other unnecessary loud distractions.
- Less or no engaging in discussions or debates or spending lots of time on the phone.
- Fill all your hours with gratitude, tons and tons of it.

In other words, go inward. Shut out the outside world. Let the Detox & Cleanse be not just for your body, but also your mind, your heart, and your soul, and let it work. Let this be a holistic cleansing, and you will emerge as a new person.

Tracy Russell

Favorite Recipe: Banana Pineapple Blast

8 ounces of almond milk
1 small banana
1 cup pineapple
2 stalks of celery
2 cups of kale, stems removed

By the time she reached her early twenties, Tracy had higher-than-normal cholesterol, difficulty managing her weight, chronic acne, and frequent heartburn. She tried a variety of diets, supplements, and health programs, but was never able to stick to them long-term because she never truly got the results she was looking for. And none of these diets were sustainable. Once she stopped dieting, she gained all the weight back. Everything came to a head after she got married and upon arriving home from her honeymoon, she weighed in at 147 pounds! It was the most she had ever weighed. She discovered green smoothies back in 2008 as a way to lose weight without feeling like she was on a diet for the rest of her life. They helped her lose forty pounds, lower her cholesterol by forty points, and she no longer gets heartburn. She also found the energy to run her first marathon! She drinks two thirty-two-ounce green smoothies a day and looks and feels better now than she did when she was in her twenties! She started IncredibleSmoothies. com in 2009 to help other people achieve the same success.

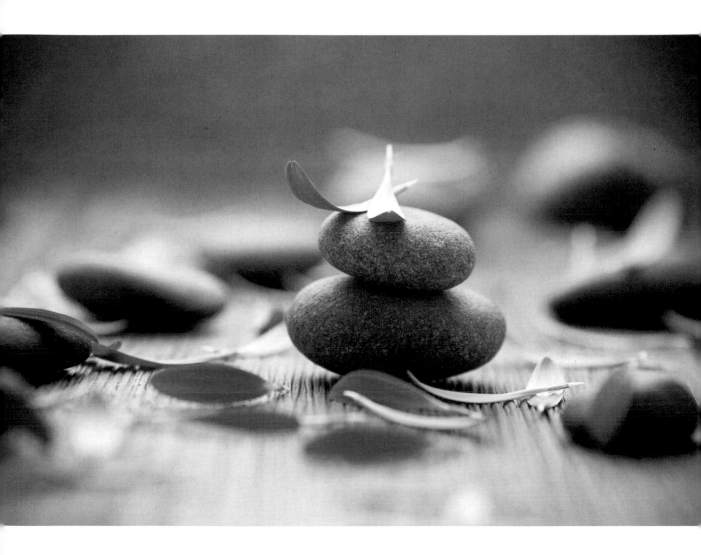

The Healthy Smoothie Lifestyle: Building the Habit

Time and health are two precious assets that we do not recognize and appreciate until they are depleted.
~Denis Whitley

If you could do something just once and get results for a lifetime, it would not be called a habit. It would be magic! A habit is something you do regularly, and then the power of consistency builds momentum and carries you forward until it becomes second nature. Habits can change your life and keep you attached at the hip to those health goals. Habits are your shield against procrastination, inconsistency, irregularity, and laziness. Habits are your friend, and your smoothie habit can even become your best friend.

Habits can also be fun to establish. Who knew? I'm going to give you my best tips and shortcuts to getting your smoothie habit down pat. Ready to do this?

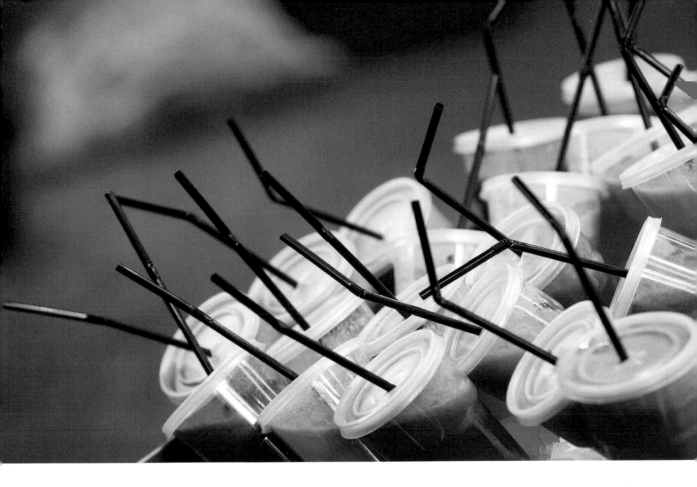

Improvise Your Own Smoothies

To insure good health: eat lightly, breathe deeply, live moderately, cultivate cheer-fulness, and maintain an interest in life.
~William Londen

As you are building your smoothie habit, be open to experimenting and improvising. In other words, be willing to play and get creative and make smoothies your way. The goal is not to find one perfect smoothie that you make every day. You will get bored fast and lose enthusiasm. Plus, you now know it's important to rotate your greens and not use the same old bunch of spinach in every green smoothie. There is no one single recipe that will have all your daily nutritional recommendations, but you can find several that together will give you a balanced and delicious powerhouse of nutrition. The goal is also not to pick a super healthy smoothie that you can't stand and force yourself to gulp it down. The idea is to find the right combinations that work for your taste buds while giving you tons of nutrients and energy.

You do not have to sacrifice taste for nutrition when it comes to healthy smoothies. That's the beauty of it. The way the food blends together, you can create a super food that tastes wonderful and is extremely good for you, and there are endless combinations so continue experimenting. There are over 100 recipes in this book to give you ideas on how different combinations create new flavors, so that eventually you can become a master at creating your own smoothies.

Your Smoothie, Your Way

You are the boss of you in all areas of your life, and your smoothies should be no exception. All that you read here in this book or any other book is a guideline to help get you started. There are no rules or laws about how thick or thin a smoothie should be, or whether it should be drunk through a straw or eaten with a spoon. I personally like thick, creamy smoothies, and I love using a spoon on occasion and feel like I am "eating my breakfast" instead of just drinking it. You can use a straw or spoon for your smoothie. My hubby and I have actually debated over this. If you are spooning it out, is it still a smoothie? (I say yes!) Since your smoothies will come out in varying consistencies, you make the call. You may want to drink it out of your cup, or use a straw (glass or disposable), or have a spoon and enjoy your thick smoothie that way. Your smoothie, your way! Got it?

If the recipes in the book yield thicker smoothies than you like, thin it out with water. You can add up to ½ cup of water to any recipe in this book and hardly mess up the taste, yet a little water can improve the consistency and cut down bitterness or sweetness. This is a quick and easy fix to any smoothie that's not exactly your way.

Is It Really All Too Simple?

The whole point of making smoothies a health habit is because they are simple, quick, and easy. Sure, you can get fancy and make a fun complex smoothie with fifteen ingredients and so many flavors that you don't get the same taste on any two sips. But you can just as easily "Keep It Simple, Baby," especially as you start to create your own.

Simplicity is one of the reasons you are turning to smoothies, and all you need for a healthy smoothie is some fruit, a handful of greens, and a liquid base, and off you go. You're done! That's your basic foundation for a healthy, super nutritious smoothie.

To help you get started on improvising your own smoothie, here are some three-ingredient smoothie combinations that work well. Use these combinations to build out your first dozen simple smoothies. Remember, you still get to add a liquid base.

Fruit + Fruit + Fruit
Fruit + Fruit + Green
Fruit + Vegetable + Green
Fruit + Green + Green
Vegetable + Vegetable + Green
Vegetable + Green + Green

I would not go green all the way, and I'd always choose a vegetable that adds some sweetness, such as carrot and tomato, when you are mixing it with two other greens.

You can also add a squirt of lemon or lime—it's okay, we won't count this one as a fourth ingredient—and use filtered water or your favorite unsweetened nut milk as base. If your fruit isn't frozen, add some ice.

As far as ratios, here's a rough estimate that works well: Use one quantity, or half, depending on the size if the fruit or vegetable is countable, such as one mango, one (small) avocado, one banana (but of course, not one whole pineapple). When a fruit has more than one serving, use one cup of it. For the greens, go for one to two handfuls, or two loosely packed cups.

Here are some excellent trio combinations all using filtered water as a liquid base:
Spinach + Banana + any Berry
Spinach + Mango + Orange
Spinach + Avocado + Apple or Pear
Spinach + Parsley + Apple (with a dash of lemon or lime)
Spinach + Parsley + Pineapple
Kale + Banana + any Berry
Kale + Avocado + Pineapple (with small chunk of ginger)
Swiss chard + Banana + Orange
Swiss chard + Mango + any Berry
Swiss chard + Cucumber + Tomato (savory, can add garlic, a dash of sea salt, lemon or lime)

If you want to use almond or other nut milk as base for any smoothie, you can do that, too. I love using water for all savory recipes. Learn to create water-based recipes that you can also use during Detox & Cleanse regimens.

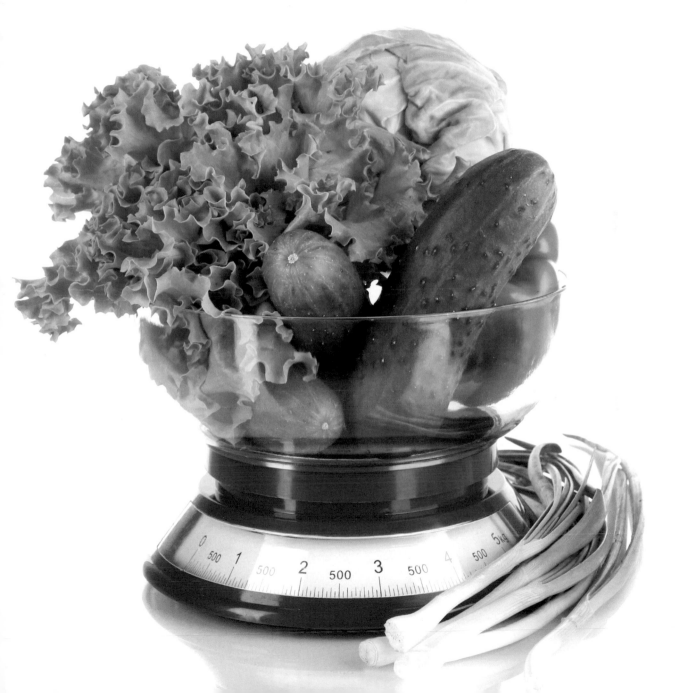

If you get tired of using banana as a creamy sweet base, then I would recommend replacing it with an avocado for creaminess, followed by a handful of grapes or a couple of pitted dates for sweetness. You can safely make this replacement with some change in the overall taste of the smoothie naturally. You can also replace frozen banana for frozen mango or papaya to get that creamy sweet taste. In addition, you will notice soaked oats as well as nut butters in the recipes in this book. You can use them for the creamy consistency also.

You get the idea. Experiment with simple three-ingredient recipes and get the hang of how the combinations work. Then you can move on to adding more goodies to your delicious concoctions.

Five Compelling Reasons to Keep Your Smoothies Simple

1. Pure fresh fruits and vegetables blended are easiest and gentlest on your digestive system.
2. The raw, natural, fresh foods, without anything powdered or bottled, are the highest value in nutrition.
3. Keeping it only to fruits and vegetables is the most budget-friendly option.
4. Simple smoothies are the fastest meals you can whip up in nearly no time.
5. Enhances your taste buds and appreciation of raw whole fruits and vegetables at their purest.

Of course you can—but do not necessarily need to—make it more fun and complex by adding nuts, seeds, nut butters, protein powders, superfoods, unsweetened dried fruits, and supplements to enhance the nutrition and up the filling factor of your smoothie.

When should you add the extra "stuff" and when should you keep it simple? Well, a mix of your whole fruits, fresh vegetables, and greens yields the best superfood, so add extra if you feel you need something beyond this fantastic base.

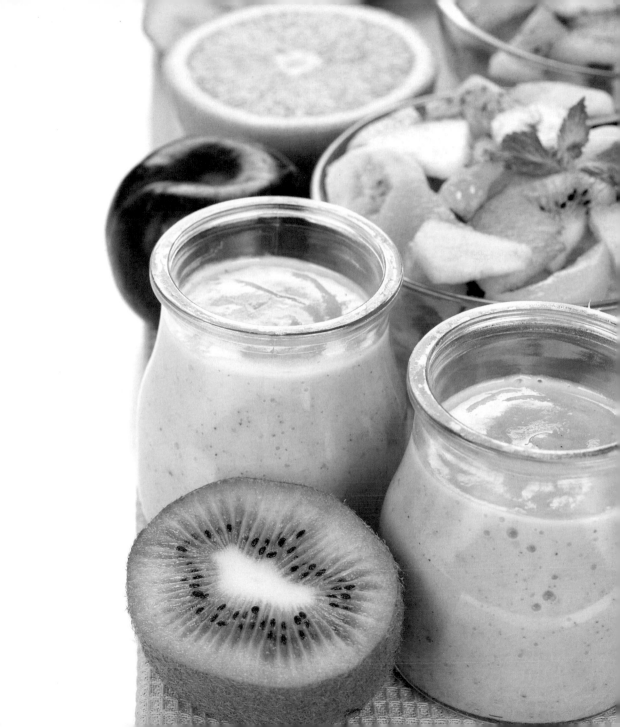

My advice to you is to keep your recipes simple, especially as you are starting out and getting familiar with new greens or new food combinations that you haven't had before. I have a very sensitive stomach, and there have been several occasions when a smoothie gave me a stomachache for hours. I had mixed so many different items, I had no idea which was the culprit, but it's also possible that the resulting complicated taste did not go over well with me. Adding too much fat with nuts and omega-3 fatty acids to a green smoothie can affect digestion, cause gas and bloating, and even affect your blood sugar, so go easy on these ingredients.

Whenever I simplify, I get great results. Start simple, with only three to maximum five ingredients, plus your base liquid. Simple is better, especially as you are starting out. Don't feel you need to "protein-load" or "nutrient-load" your meals. Nature provides the right amount of nutrients in fruit and vegetables. As long as you eat enough calories each day, you should do well without needing to artificially "enhance" your green smoothies.

Now there are some good reasons to (slowly) add complexity to your smoothie. Once you get the hang of the simple smoothie ingredients and which ones work well for your body and your cravings, you may want to add more "stuff" on occasion. Here's three reasons you may want to add superfoods and spices to your smoothie:

1. You want it as a meal replacement with additional proteins, fats, and higher-calorie ingredients to keep you full for longer.
2. You want to "hide" your supplements such as your daily dose of omega-3s and other vitamins, if you are not getting these in your regular diet.
3. You want to spice it up and have fun with the superfoods and create new recipes.

So if you are in a hurry, and you are making a smoothie as a quick healthy snack, rather than a whole meal replacement, then keep it simple. Make sure the rest of your diet is providing you with enough calories, fats, and proteins, so you don't rely on the smoothie for all that. But if you are using the smoothie as a meal replacement, and plan to go a few hours before eating again, then feel free to add a protein boost, some healthy fats, and other nutritious boosts to make it more of a complete meal.

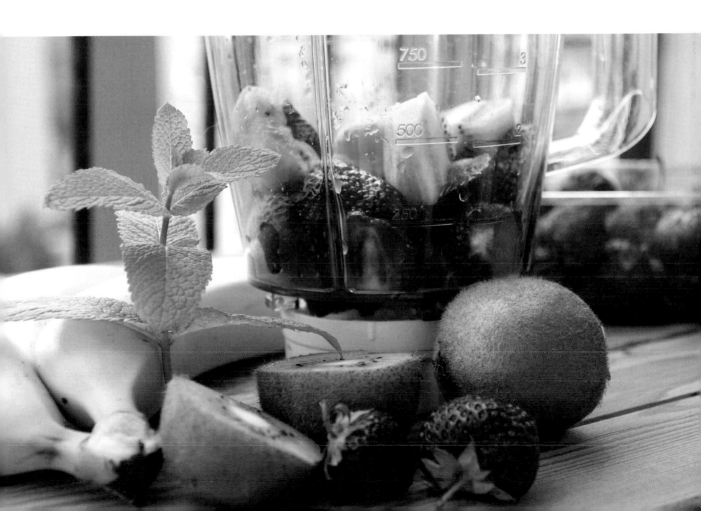

Building the Smoothie Habit

Health and understanding are the two great blessings of life.
~Greek Proverb

A health habit is something you do regularly because it makes you feel good and gives you some health benefits. Building a smoothie habit is no different. It makes you feel really good. Plus you enjoy the many benefits that I outlined earlier. You will detox and cleanse your body with delicious smoothies, trim down to your ideal weight, adjust your bad cravings, feel confident and sexy in your body, skyrocket your natural energy, develop a stronger immune system against common colds and flu, and understand how to make positive changes in your life by starting where it matters the most: your body, your temple.

Most basic and effective rule for establishing a habit: Start simple but start now.

Starting is often the hardest step. We think about it and analyze it way too much. Just tell yourself you will start having one green smoothie a day starting Monday. Then work backwards to make it happen. But it can be challenging even then, I really get it. So in this section, I want to help you establish mini-regimens to get you started and established with your green smoothie and healthy smoothie habit.

With every health habit, you have a choice. You can look at it as something to do and get over and done with. Or you can look at it as a journey, an experience, a path that teaches you more about who you are, what your likes and tolerances are, and how willing you are to explore new things and grow to become a better version of yourself in the process. So let your healthy smoothies be a *big deal*, take it seriously, and make it a mission to build this habit in your life. It will do your body heaps of good.

One guideline for targeting a good mix of recipes for your habit as you are starting out is to follow the 4x4x4 guideline: Every month, identify twelve different smoothie recipes made from a menu of four types of greens, four types of vegetables, and four different fruits. As a bonus, choose the ones that also have some healthy fats, such as avocado or flaxseed powder or chia seeds. This arrangement makes it possible for you to shop relatively easily for all the ingredients without getting overwhelmed, get enough variety to rotate your veggies for excellent overall nutrition, and also create some distinct-tasting smoothies. As you go through the recipes in this book, mark the ones that taste good and meet these criteria.

Here are my favorite 4x4x4 combinations:

Four vegetables:

Celery
Avocado
Cucumber
Broccoli

Four greens:

Spinach
Kale
Parsley
Swiss chard

Four fruits:

Orange
Banana
Berries (any kind)
Pear

For each recipe, I would choose one vegetable, one green, and up to two fruits. You can skip a vegetable or a green, but try to have at least one of them in your smoothie, if possible. If you want to stick to all fruit at first, pick three or four fruits.

For example, here are sample recipes from the above 4x4x4 combination:

Recipe #1: 1 stalk celery, 1 cup spinach, 1 orange, 1 cup berries.
Recipe #2: ½ avocado, 2 large leaves of kale (no stem), 1 orange (peeled), ½ banana.
Recipe #3: 1 cucumber, 1 handful parsley, ½ pear, 1 frozen banana.

After you select your 4x4x4, you can create dozens of recipes. But all you need for your first month is one dozen. Choose the dozen and rotate them. You could do recipes one, two, and three in week one; recipes four, five, and six in week two; recipes seven, eight, and nine in week three; and recipes ten, eleven, and twelve in week four. Each week, you have three recipes to play with, and if you make more than three smoothies that week, you can make the same one twice. This will significantly simplify your shopping and still give you plenty of variety and fun. It will also help you with a system to build your habit.

Drinking your smoothie:

Take your time drinking the smoothie. You don't have to gulp it down in thirty seconds (not that I've done that or anything!). Instead, enjoy every sip. Take it to work or have it at your work desk at home, or enjoy it during your commute, and remind yourself to slow down, enjoy every sip, and remember that you are doing your body such good! Plus this way, you feel nice and satisfied without filling up too fast.

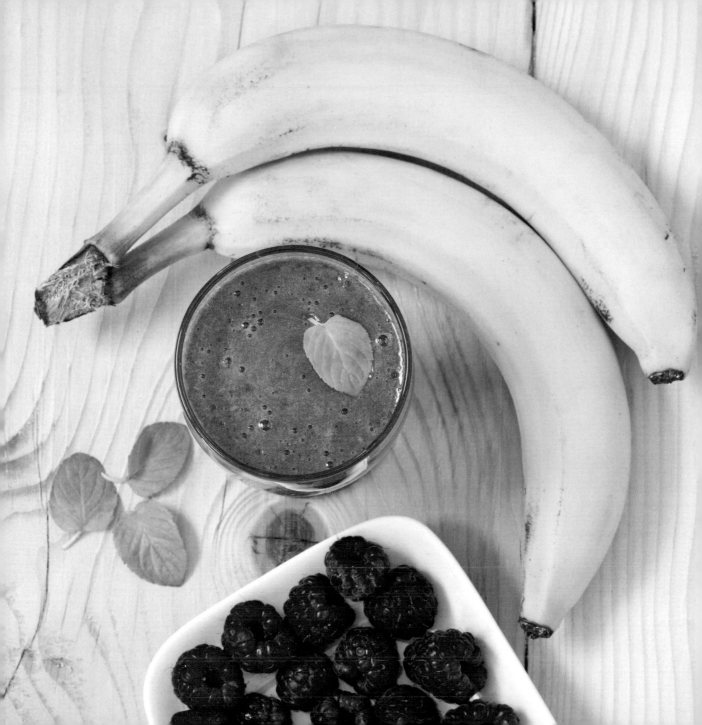

Should You Survive Just On Smoothies?

No. Absolutely not. You should not give up solid food permanently for smoothies. The idea here is not to go replacing all your meals, no matter how excited you may be about smoothies. Your body needs a variety of nutrition and if nothing else, you need solid foods to keep your jaws strong and your teeth in tip top condition through the act of regular chewing and to keep your digestive system working efficiently.

While green smoothies can be a fantastic foundation for your health, they are far from the *only* nourishment your body needs. Instead of giving up the rest of your food and feeling deprived for no good reason, a better goal is to simply become more aware of what you put in your body. Smoothies help you to do that by gently enhancing your cravings and fine-tuning your taste buds. These healthy nutrient-rich drinks act as a gateway to better health and to more raw foods. They help calm down your lust for processed sugar by showing you a better way to manage your sweet tooth. They also open your mind to a world of new tastes that you did not know before—new fruits, new vegetables, new greens and herbs, and other superfoods—and this fresh new excitement for your palate is the best way to wean off the bad cravings and delve more into healthy, unprocessed whole foods.

The benefits you get from adding smoothies naturally into a healthy diet is far better than any benefits you may get from consuming *just* smoothies all day long.

How Often Should You Make a Smoothie?

When you are first starting out, one smoothie a day, three times a week is a great frequency. If you can swing it four to five times a week, even better. This is a nice way to ease into your smoothie regimen and find your groove. You can choose any healthy smoothies (green or not), but focus on keeping up the consistency. It is better to be consistent with a three-times-a-week regimen for two months than to make ten smoothies the first week and then not touch the blender for two more weeks! Consistency is your friend, and it is the way to adjust your taste buds, build the habit, and make smoothies a part of your regular diet.

For instance, with consistency, if smoothies serve as your 3:00 p.m. snack as you build them into your regular schedule, you come to expect and crave them, and perhaps even replace the afternoon cup of coffee or cookie with this new healthy drink. Your body's clock begins to whisper: *"Give me a smoothie at 3:00 p.m., please"* instead of *"I need a cuppa coffee or I'm going to collapse!"* But if you are not consistent about it long enough to build the habit, which is about four weeks on average, then you throw off the cycle and confuse your body with mixed signals. If you don't build a solid foundation for your new habit, you may return to your old cravings. But if you stick with it and follow a regimen for one to two months, your body will crave the smoothie over other junk food and find it plenty sweet for your afternoon "sugar rush."

I like to think of myself as a big sweet onion. Every health journey helps me peel off a layer and get closer to my core, to my true self. I feel like I am shedding old skin and replenishing with new, fresh skin every time I do a detox or take better care of myself. Imagery keeps me focused on the why behind the habit. Feel free to steal my imagery or come up with your own relevant to your present state and your desired goals on this journey. The idea is to make it easy to remind yourself why you are doing this, what's in it for you, and why it's so important that you continue your smoothie habit, as you would your flossing habit or hair-brushing habit. Before you know it, it becomes a daily ritual!

Smoothie Habit Building Challenges

I put together these series of challenges to help you build a smoothie habit into your life. This is not the same as the detox regimen in the previous section. Here, you are simply

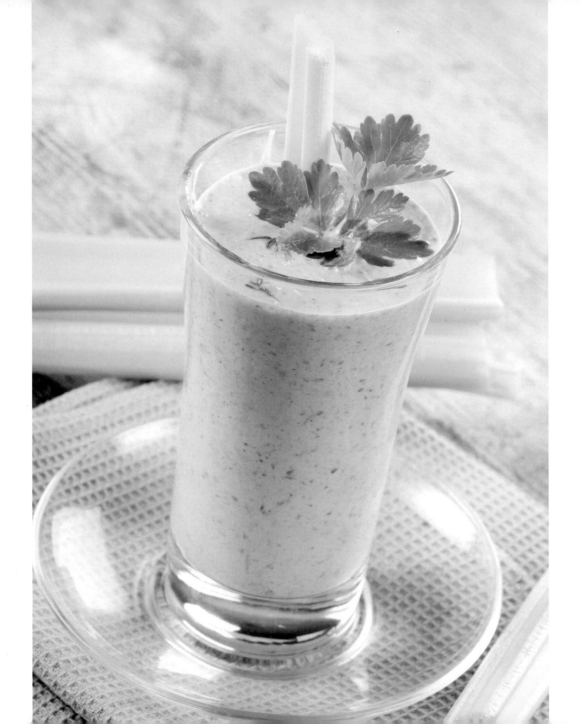

building the consistent habit of making smoothies into your lifestyle. As a result, you may very well enjoy some benefits of detox, but detox and cleanse is not the main goal here.

If you want to incorporate smoothies slowly into your life, follow these three challenges. The challenge here is great if you have a really busy lifestyle and a lot of commitments around eating with others and little time to yourself in your kitchen.

- Do a three-day smoothie as a breakfast or snack challenge
- Take a minimum one- to two-day / maximum one-week break from smoothies
- Do a seven-day smoothie for one meal per day challenge
- Take a minimum one- to two-day / maximum one-week break from smoothies
- Do a twenty-one-day, one smoothie a day minimum, and up to two smoothies a day challenge

Each smoothie should be at least ten to twelve ounces, but you can have a larger portion. Don't go over twenty-four ounces per day when you are first starting the challenge. After you finish all three challenges, you'll feel the craving for the (almost) daily smoothie. If you miss a day in your challenge, continue on without beating yourself up. As long as you keep going after you fall off the challenge, you are going to build this habit for life.

If you like intensity and can't wait to start your smoothie habit, double the length of the days in the above challenge and take shorter breaks. Here's a modified regimen below. This challenge is more intense and gives you a chance to try a variety of recipes, replace one meal for a smoothie per day, and get your body habituated to the idea of a daily smoothie.

- Do a seven-day smoothie as breakfast or snack challenge
- Take a one- to two-day break
- Do a fourteen-day smoothie for one meal per day and up to two smoothies a day challenge

- Take a one- to two-day break
- Do a twenty-one-day, one smoothie a day minimum, and up to two smoothies a day challenge

By the end of this set of challenges, you should be hooked on smoothies and your body will crave them if you go so much as a day without them. This is the way to make habits stick, when you have a natural tendency in their direction rather than using self-discipline or punishment to make yourself do something. Enjoy the process!

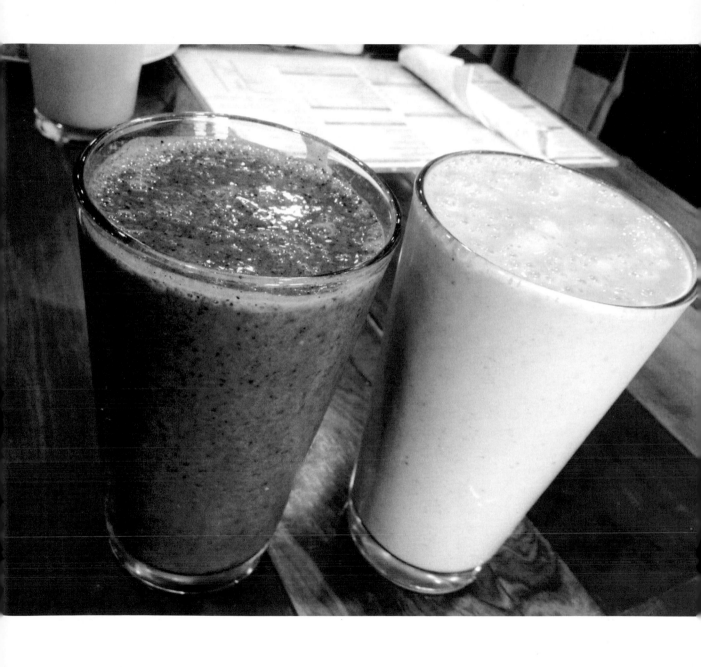

Jennifer Thompson

Favorite Recipe: Immune Booster Green Smoothie (serves 2)

1 handful fresh spinach
1 handful fresh parsley
1 banana
1 apple
1 tbsp ground flaxseed
1 tsp spirulina powder
Juice of 1 lemon
½ inch fresh ginger
Dash of organic cinnamon powder
2 cups water

Jennifer's journey into green smoothies started several years ago. Back then, she was already eating a raw food diet and drinking fresh juices, but wasn't really using a blender or making any smoothies, let alone green smoothies. After hearing all the "green smoothie" buzz, she thought, "How could this green-colored muck actually taste good?" and had to try it for herself to see. She bought some fruit and greens and blended her very first green smoothie. That day, her energy levels soared. The next day, she noticed how much faster she ran, and over the course of a week of having a daily green smoothie, she saw her skin get even clearer and look more youthful, and the whites of her eyes even got brighter. People were asking her if she was on a juice fast because she looked so good. She would tell them, "No! I'm just drinking one green smoothie a day!" Six months later, she started teaching green smoothie classes from her own kitchen at home, and seven years later, she made her first DVD, *Green Smoothie Power.* What she learned in all that time is this: Even if you don't make any other change to your diet or lifestyle, you can and will start feeling better by drinking just one green smoothie per day. It's all in the power of the greens!

Jennifer is a fully trained and qualified IIPA-Certified Comprehensive Iridologist (CCI) and provides Iridology readings and raw food coaching to clients; teaches raw food and healthy living courses; offers detox, fasting, and cleansing support; and gives motivational lectures to educate and inspire others on their journey of healing. You can find her at healthybliss.net.

Closing Words & Best Wishes for Blending

It is health that is real wealth and not pieces of gold and silver.
~Mahatma Gandhi

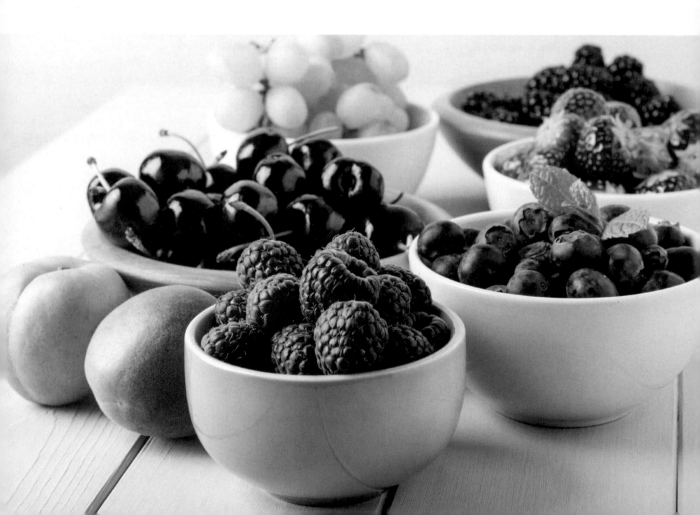

We started this book with one simple idea: how to fall in love with fruits, greens, vegetables, and healthy smoothies, and I want to close on that note because loving what you put in your body is the easiest and best way to maintain the health habit for life.

Any step you take, starting tomorrow, toward building your smoothie habit counts. Getting your kitchen ready counts as one step. Buying the right blender and setting up your smoothie station counts as the next step. Preparing yourself mentally and emotionally, as well as announcing this new upcoming change to your family, counts as yet another step. Whether they participate or not is not as important right now as it is for you to get started right away. Become the model that they will want to follow, rather than forcing them into drinking that glass of green concoction because "it's good for you!" The gentle invitation to a healthy smoothie goes much further, and if you really want to get your family members onboard, just let them drive. Help them come up with a fun recipe and give them all the credit for it. Make it look like this whole thing was their idea, and they will be inspiring you as much as you are them to make this a non-negotiable part of your lifestyle.

The most important things to keep in mind are to experiment and to be open to new tastes. If you don't like a particular fruit or vegetable, don't rule it out. Be open to the idea of adding it into a smoothie. You may not even taste it, or you may be surprised with how the blended taste is totally different from the standalone taste. If you have reservations about a new green, then make a small batch first. That way you don't waste a lot of ingredients, and you get to find out for a fact how that new green tastes when mixed with other ingredients. Give yourself permission to be creative after you get the hang of basic healthy smoothies. You get to play with a lot of ingredients in this book, but by no means did I use all of the fruits, vegetables, nuts, seeds, and greens that you can use in a smoothie. Before you know it, you'll be teaching someone else how to make the perfect green smoothie using your best practices!

So where does the love come in? Maybe you have noticed it by the time you read this section. If not, you've got something great to look forward to. As you drink healthy and especially green smoothies, you will begin to notice a change in your relationship with food. You will look at celery and spinach and apples differently. You will have a relationship with parsley and never look at bananas and avocados the same way. You will be in love, I'm telling you.

Before you know it, you will be coming up with recipes in your head, schemes to freeze that new fruit you just spotted for the next smoothie, and wondering how mixing such and such together will taste in your blender. You'll go through your days making a mental note to take in all your nutrients in a glass of smoothie, and you'll reach for the blender as soon as you feel the onset of a cold or flu because you know the magic to fight it off fast is in these wonderful, beautiful whole foods that are never far out of reach.

Most of all, you will learn how to tune into your body, how to listen to your true desires, and how to identify and respond to emotional food cravings versus real ones. When this happens, you'll be in charge of your health, your body, and your beautiful future. When this happens, you'll feel the love.

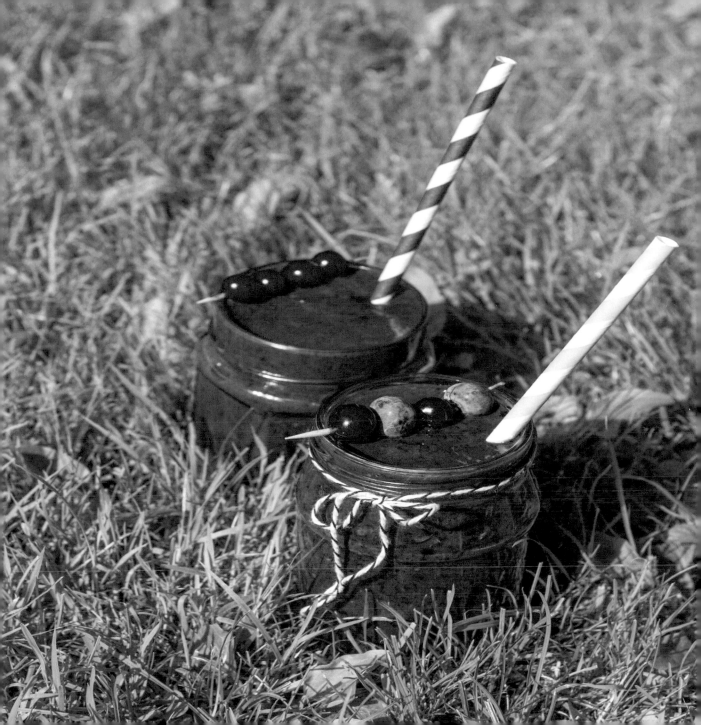

Recipe Index

Top Brand Product Recommendations and Gratitude

The author would like to acknowledge the generosity of the companies listed below for providing samples to test in her recipes, and for their mission to help create a healthier, cleaner world for us through better nutrition:

Standard Process
www.standardprocess.com

Vega
www.myvega.com

Amazing Grass
www.amazinggrass.com

PlantFusion
www.plantfusion.net

Sunwarrior
www.sunwarrior.com

Onnit
www.onnit.com

Miessence
www.miessence.com

Raw Power
www.rawpower.com

Manitoba Harvest
www.manitobaharvest.com

Living Harvest
www.livingharvest.com

Navitas Naturals
www.navitasnaturals.com

Green Life Foods
www.greenlifefoods.net

Nutrex Hawaii

www.nutrex-hawaii.com

Ingredients and Highlights Index

Throughout this index, page numbers in italics refer to recipes.

cucumber, 50, 57, *141, 143, 145, 152,*
185, 186, 192, 198, 207, 233

D

Dairy Free SP Complete protein
powder, *158*
dairy-free, 37–39
dandelion, 55, 128, *155, 183, 185,*
188, 192
dates, 98, 115, 126, *176, 183, 185,*
188, 191, 197, 199, 201, 204
Detox & Cleanse
activities, suggestions for, 219
benefits of, 24, 211, 212, 218–219
caffeine intake and, 214–215, 216
defined, 211
foods to avoid in, 215
healthy smoothies and, 210, 211,
212, 213–215
how it works, 212
initial symptoms, and side effects,
211, 217–218
introduction to, 210
smoothies, 133
suggested regimens, 216
tips for successful, 216
what to consume, 213–215
what to expect, and modifying as
needed, 217–218
diets, 15–16, 30

F

Farnoosh's Signature Gems, 133
fasting, 32, 211
Fat Loss Fundamentals (Cooper), 51
fennel, 58, *147, 190, 192, 201*
fiber, 25, 28, 32, 42, 51, 61, 72, 124,
212
figs, 63, 66, 87, 106, 108, 126, *161,*

162, 164, 165, 167, 171
filtered water, 80, 81. *see also* water-
based smoothies
flaxseed powder, 71, 72–73, 76, 77,
79, *152, 156, 161, 165, 167, 175,*
176, 180, 183, 185, 196, 202, 234,
242
Food & Drug Administration (FDA),
49
food processors, 97
freezing food
fruit, 35, 39, 47
greens and, 53
prepared smoothie, 119
tips for successful, 104–107
when not to, 64
fruit
as bases and flavors, 63, 84–86,
225–226, 228
digestive process and, 212
foundations, and creating
smoothies, 47, 225–226, 233–
234
freezing tips, 104–107
fresh use only, 104
measurement in recipes, 128
mixing and matching flavors, 53,
84–86
store-bought frozen, 109
top twenty choices for smoothies,
64–68

G

garlic, 61, 115, *184, 185, 193*
ginger, 61, *138, 140, 141, 143, 145,*
147, 153, 155, 159, 172, 175, 192,
197, 242
gluten-free concerns, 30, 73, 124
goji berries, 70, 72, 77, *157, 160,*
162–163, 190, 206

grapes, 64, *138, 159, 165*
Green Lover Recipes, 132
Green Smoothie Power (DVD), 243
green smoothies
benefits of, 120, 242–243
daily nutritional requirements and,
25–26
foundation basics, 225–226
fruit additions, 84
green powders, 61
"Hidden Greens" recipes, 132
ingredients in
adding fats to, 230
guidelines, 52
measurement in recipes, 226
rotating types of, 53, 223
top ten choices, 34–36. *see also*
specific greens
low sugar content as starting
point, 42
for optimum nutrition, 35, 47–48
overcoming aversion to idea of,
49–50, 126
produce preparation
storing, 99
washing, 100
recipes from contributors. *see also*
Recipe Index
Blended Salad Smoothie,
50–51
Citrus Breeze, *120*
Immune Booster Green
Smoothie, *242*
Key Lime Pie Green Thickie,
98
Tropical Pineapple Dream, *36*
superfoods and, 70–71, 92
using in recipes, 128, 130
and weight loss, 27

53, 84–86, 224–225
simplify, five reasons to, 226,
228, 230
trio combinations and ratios,
225–226
juices versus, 32–34, 35
meal replacement, 43–45, 50–51,
230, 231, 240, 240–241
problems, fixing, 114–115, 130,
224–225
snack smoothies, 43–45, 231, 237,
240–241
soaking nuts, seeds, and oats,
110–112
storing, 118–119
texture and consistency, 117,
223–224
solid food, 16, 51, 115, 216, 236
soy products, 38, 79, 81
spices, 61, 85, 115, *155, 181. see also
specific spices*
spinach, 36, 54, 55, 79, *88, 98, 120,
136, 138, 140, 143, 144, 146, 147,
150, 152, 153, 154, 155, 157, 158,
161, 162, 164, 165, 167, 168, 171,
172, 173, 175, 176, 180, 183, 185,
188, 190, 191, 195, 196, 197, 204,
206,* 226, 233, *242*
spirulina, 74–75, 77, 79, *194, 197,
206, 242*
Standard Process Protein Powder, *200*
strawberries, 64, 79, *88, 138, 139,
141, 148, 149, 157, 159, 165, 177,
179, 183, 191, 194, 196, 197, 198,
199, 200*
sugars/sweeteners
avoiding, 22, 47, 87
in commercial products, 34–35
cravings for, controlling, 18, 64, 87
fructose, versus processed sugars,
40–42, 47, 87
in fruit, 40–42

natural, 87
sunflower seeds, 74, 98, *159, 186, 193*
superfoods. *see also* acai berry powder;
cacao powder, raw; chia seeds/
powder; goji berries; hemp seeds/
powder; matcha green tea; sesame
seeds; spirulina; sunflower seeds
brands recommended, 77–78,
252–253
buying, 92
overview of, 70–72
in recipes, *161, 166*
types of, 61, 72–75
sweet potato, 58, *181*
swiss chard, 55, *137, 141, 169, 171,
172, 190, 196, 201, 202, 204, 205,*
226, 233

T

The Healthy Juicer's Bible (Brock), 35,
211
Thompson, Jennifer, 242–243
tomatoes, 58, *184, 185, 186, 193*
toxin avoidance, 53. *see also* Detox &
Cleanse

V

vanilla, 85, *179, 180, 189, 191*
vanilla almond milk, *69, 154, 162*
vanilla protein powder/meal
replacement, *148, 153*
vegan diet, 20, 24, 30, 35, 73, 76, 124
vegetables, 57–59, 233
vegetarian diet, 20, 30, 79
Velasquez, Vickie, 79
Vitamix blender, 32, 93, 95, 96, 117

W

Waldman, Joshua, 36
walnuts, 110, *136–137, 143*

warranties, 95
water-based smoothies, *36, 120,
136, 137, 138, 139, 140, 141, 143,
144, 145, 146–147, 150, 152, 153,
154, 155, 158, 159, 168, 171–172,
180, 182, 183, 184–185, 186, 190,
192–193, 196, 197, 200, 201, 202,
204, 207,* 226, *242*
websites. *see* blogs and websites of
interest
weight loss, 27, 44, 133, 148, 220
workout food, 28, 73, 79

Y

yogurt, 37, 38